Brain Injury Targets
Individuals

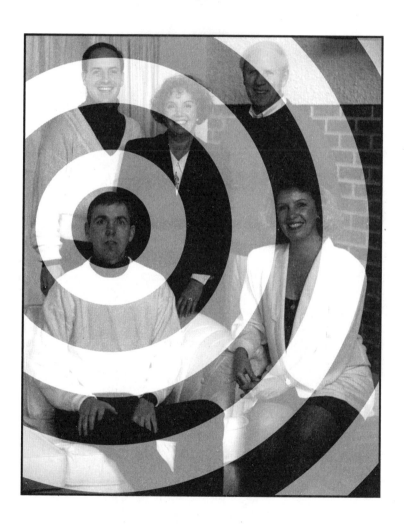

But Happens to Families

ver Photo by: Lee's Studio, Escanaba, Michigan
ver Design Concept by: Jeffery Abrahamson

BRAIN INJURY: A FAMILY TRAGEDY

Patt Abrahamson
with
Jeffery Abrahamson

HDI Publishers
Houston, Texas

HDI Publishers
P.O. Box 131401
Houston, Texas 77219
Toll free (800) 321-7037
Tel (713) 682-8700
Fax (713) 956-2288

Printed in the United States of America.

This book is printed on acid-free paper. ∞

Abrahamson, Patt, 1933-
    Brain injury : a family tragedy / Patt Abrahamson, with Jeffery
Abrahamson.
        p.   cm.
    ISBN 1-882855-56-6 (alk. paper)
    1. Abrahamson, Gary--Health. 2. Brain damage--Patients--
United States--Biography. 3. Brain damage--Patients--United
States--Family relationships. I. Abrahamson, Gary. II.
Abrahamson, Jeffery, 1958-   . III. Title
RC387.5.A26A27   1997
362.1'968'0092--dc21
[B]   97-11774
                                                              CIP

DEDICATION

To my son, Gary — the Gary before his brain injury as well as the Gary after his brain injury, both of whom I love and accept — whose tragic destiny and our family's attempt to deal with it is the subject of this book.

To Gary's father and my husband, Gary Senior, who has given his enduring love, support, and fellowship — through good times and bad — to help form the partnership we have today, without which this book would not have been written.

To the rest of my family — my son Jeff, his wife Peggy, my daughter Vicki Cass, her husband Dave. To my grandchildren from those marriages — Heather, Graham, Zachary, and Mary Pat; and to my great-grandchild Gabrielle.

And to Gary's children, Arlo and Leif, in the hope that one day they will heal from the loss of their father as they knew him and will come to honor and accept him as he is today.

CONTENTS

ACKNOWLEDGEMENTS

I would like to acknowledge the support of my youngest son, Jeffery Abrahamson, who managed to find time to help me while also tending to his family, work, and evening law school. His dedication, expert help, and contacts in Washington, D.C. proved to be of invaluable assistance to me. I particularly want to thank him for his service and creativity during the final writing and editing process; he helped develop my ideas, organize my thoughts, and polish my prose. Although I was the object of his efforts, the primary beneficiary will be the reader, who will find this book more readable and interesting.

A special thanks also goes to Norma Bauer, who was not only instrumental in encouraging me to write this story but displayed faith all along the way that it would eventually be published. Norma, with whom I collaborated on certain words or phrases, not only typed and re-typed the manuscript but provided helpful suggestions in marketing the book to publishers.

Finally, I would like to thank Lorelei Kornell for her service, Alan Howard and John Porter for their contributions and encouragement, and HDI Publishers' J. Charles Haynes, who appreciated the need to publish a book about family survival after brain injury.

- PATT ABRAHAMSON

Caring for my brother Gary is a giant undertaking, so I was a bit surprised when my mother informed me that she was going to write a book. But, then, I was surprised when she began college at age 55 and received a bachelor's degree with honors at age 59. More recently, I was again surprised to hear that she won the Ms. Senior Michigan 1997 pageant. What is most surprising is that she did all of this while caring for my brother after his brain injury!

Mom, please forgive me — I will stop being surprised by you; but what you have been able to accomplish in the face of apparent adversity is admirable. The best of luck to you in the Ms. Senior America pageant.

Collaborating on this book was a labor of love. Thank you for the opportunity. I only hope that those who come to read it — particularly those who never really knew Gary, including my wife and daughter — will gain insight into the person he was, the brother, husband, and father he was, the brother-in-law or uncle he could have been, rather than the hapless, tragic person he has become.

Writing a book, seeing it published — that's gratifying. But I regret that the writing of this book was occasioned by my brother's brain injury; I would, of course, rather have my brother back. For this reason, writing this book has, for me, produced distinctly mixed sensations — sort of like a silvery-scaled fish that has washed ashore; it has a dazzling shine when light is reflected on it, yet its inhospitable bouquet leaves you wanting.

- JEFFERY ABRAHAMSON

PREFACE

After a jog, stretching in his front yard, my son Gary collapsed and died. He had no respiration, no heart beat. Medical technology was able to snatch him from the throes of death, but not before oxygen deprivation robbed him of his very being, the essence of who he was.

From a coma, he emerged a stranger cloaked in my son's body, lost in the abyss of amnesia, unable to remember yesterday, incapable of anticipating tomorrow. He was and is a man lost in time and space. While medical technology may have saved Gary's life, he is left with the maladies of a severe brain injury for which medical or rehabilitative treatment has, thus far, proven largely ineffective.

And it is no comfort to know that he is not alone. More than two million individuals sustain traumatic brain injuries each year. While advances in medical technology have decreased the incidence of death, it also means that relatively more individuals must live with their severe brain injuries.

The numbers are staggering. Each year produces another 1.9 million brain injury survivors, of which 100,000 are left with permanent, severe, and multiple impairments (i.e. cognitive, physical, and emotional), requiring intensive rehabilitation and long-term care and support.

My story, Gary's story, is about the life-long, tragic effects of brain injury — both on the survivor and his family. It depicts the many stresses and challenges faced by family members. And it exposes some of the shortcomings of our brain injury health care system, which not only lacks the medical knowledge for effective treatment of those with severe brain injury, but it can be impersonal, bureaucratic, and detached. Faced with scant resources and the daunting responsibility of caring for our son after his brain injury, my husband and I had to fight back when our requests for services and pleas for help were denied.

In the beginning, we felt almost as lost as Gary. Even the so-called medical and rehabilitative experts seemed at a loss or disagreed on what to do or what to expect. My main motive for writing this book is to impart our experience to families who — initially ignorant of its ramifications, its life-long consequences — must nevertheless enter the bizarre world of brain injury and learn to navigate the system.

Brain injury can happen — either from a blow to the head, a gun-shot wound, or from insufficient oxygen result-ing from a stroke, heart attack, or near-drowning — to any-one at anytime. Although a majority of brain injuries are caused by accidents, ours is a tragic story that begins with medical negligence. My son was a functional, integrated, keenly sensitive and responsive young, family man of 37 — full of hope and plans for a bright future. In a single instant, he was transformed, and so were the lives of his family and others close to him.

In the pages that follow, you will come to know a family torn apart, driven to divorce, even with thoughts of suicide. The story will candidly portray hope, disappointment, guilt, anger, upheaval, agitation, emotional pain, faith and spiritu-ality, the silly humor one adopts when coping and living with a brain injury survivor, and resolution.

Yet, somewhere along the way I realized that ours is a story not unlike that of many families in our situation. When one of their own is struck by severe brain injury, families are devastated and often have trouble dealing with the serious issues of 24-hour custodial care, rehabilitation, reformation of relationships, and financial constraints. Despite the high incidence of brain injury in this country, little has been writ-ten about the pressures that the families must face. Though none of us knew it early on, it is not unusual for a spouse to eventually leave the person, that person once considered a partner-for-life after he or she becomes severely brain injured — especially when there are still children to raise. I wish I had been given a book such as this to read shortly after my son's brain injury. I wrote this book, in part, to assist families that will have to face similar issues.

But there is an even larger, looming public issue at stake. While there has been a recent focus on improving our health care system, largely escaping media attention are the profound gaps in the health care delivery system for persons with a brain injury. Although brain injury affects far more people than AIDS, it receives far less attention. As such, this book is also an attempt to educate and help produce systemic change for brain injury victims (both current and future) and their families.

There was a stack of written material on which I was able to draw in writing this book, including journals and Gary's voluminous medical records since his brain injury. Some of these medical records — from hospitals, clinics, and other institutions — are provided for the reader at various places in the book, usually in excerpted form and with some slight grammatical changes to improve readability.

I have also made use of the many pre-trial depositions given by family members, expert medical witnesses, and others in the context of a medical malpractice lawsuit that I, as Gary's legal guardian, brought on his behalf.

The book focuses on what I consider to be the most significant aspects of our life after Gary's brain injury. While most of the book is chronological, I have taken some literary license to deviate from that when it made more sense to treat an issue topically.

I have attempted to put forth — based on my best recollection — an objective story. That said, however, some of the issues and events treated in this book are infused with subjectivity and opinion — as is every autobiography ever written — for no one is able to be totally objective about issues and events that intimately touch one's own life.

In some cases, I have had to reconstruct conversations that took place. While I am convinced that all of the dialogues are true to the spirit of the actual conversations, I cannot suggest that all of them should be regarded as verbatim.

FORWARDS

Forward by James S. Brady
Former Press Secretary to President Ronald Reagan
Brain Injury Association Vice Chairman

Imagine going out to do one of the everyday tasks of life — going to the grocery store or walking the dog — and never being able to return home to the same life that you left 15 minutes before. Brain injury occurs in an instant, but its repercussions last a lifetime. Gary Abrahamson suffered a heart attack after he went for a jog. The restriction of oxygen to his brain during the heart attack left his brain permanently damaged. Before that fateful jog, Gary was an active husband and the father of two boys. After his brain injury, Gary was confused, angry, paranoid, violent, and suicidal.

All of us who experience brain injury go through dramatic personality and cognitive changes. We cannot function at the same level at which we were accustomed and at which others expect us to function, yet we are still individuals in need of meaningful, productive lives. We still have a sense of humor, an appreciation for good food, a need for friends and a desire to bring home a paycheck — just like everybody else. Brain injury affects people in different ways, and by stereotyping us together — as many well-meaning but unaware people do — we are denied our own uniqueness.

This book, in an effort to share one family's perspective, chronicles the story of a man and the frustration, grief, and confusion he experiences. However, the emotional hurt — not to mention the physical pain — is not the end of the story. Gary's injury deeply affects him and his family financially when his insurance reaches the limit. Furthermore, he becomes more and more estranged from his wife, and they eventually divorce. Everyday interactions become excruciating for Gary; he tries four times before he successfully buys the donuts he was sent to get. He denies his condition because the truth is too painful to accept.

The affects of brain injury are like the waves resulting

from a stone being dropped into a pond. While the person with the injury sinks to the bottom before resurfacing, family and loved ones feel the pain in a rippling effect. Each day, the spouse, children, siblings, and parents of the survivor have to face a new person from the one they once knew. Each wave carries a different struggle: financial challenges, daily caretaking, the search for appropriate and effective rehabilitation, and rearranged family roles. The burden on the family is enormous.

But regret over what is lost is not the emphasis of Patt Abrahamson's tale. She shows us how the devastation of a lifetime can be used to find hope and purpose where none seemingly exists. Her extraordinary love as a mother and strength as a person triumph in the brain injury rehabilitation process. She illustrates that there is gold even at the end of a darkened rainbow. Patt's tireless efforts and endless hope prevail. Norman Cousins once called hope "the hidden ingredient in any prescription." Abrahamson reveals how hope leads to healing.

This book is a lesson for us all. Those readers who have sustained a brain injury or whose loved one has sustained a brain injury will find that this book truly resonates. Those who provide care as a professional will gain valuable insights into the survivor's and especially into the family's perspective — their frustrations, their hopes, their need for information and support. Whatever your motivation for reading *Brain Injury: A Family Tragedy*, you will be uplifted by the experience.

Washington, D.C.

Forward by Congressman James C. Greenwood (R-Pennsylvania)
U.S. House of Representatives
Traumatic Brain Injury Act Sponsor

Rene Descartes dictum, "I think, therefore I am," reflects the human experience that who we are spiritually seems largely determined by how we function mentally.

For this reason it is excruciatingly painful for the family and friends of one who has suffered traumatic brain injury to see past the altered features, halting voice and tortured thought patterns and recognize the soul of the loved one they once knew. We can only imagine the terror and isolation endured by the victims themselves.

The modern miracles of emergency medical services, medivac helicopters and surgical breakthroughs have enabled us to save the lives of those with serious brain injuries that were fatal until very recently. Now we must make certain that the lives we save are worth living.

Mothers like Patt Abrahamson and other committed family members and advocates are pioneers in restructuring our mental health, Medicaid, Social Security, and educational systems to make room and provide appropriate services for their loved ones.

Brain Injury: A Family Tragedy chronicles this journey with all its frustrations and victories. It offers a message of hope not just for others coming to grips with traumatic brain injury, but for anyone driven by love to make the world work as it should.

Washington, D.C.

Forward by George A. Zitnay, Ph.D.
President and CEO
Brain Injury Association, Inc.

Brain Injury: A Family Tragedy is must reading for clinicians, family members, and anyone interested in brain injury. Sometimes it is full of hope, other times you can almost feel the despair and frustration. At all times, however, it is a compelling story that should be read by the general public.

Many think what happened to Gary will never happen to them or to a loved one, yet over two million Americans sustain a brain injury every year — one every 15 seconds. Brain injury *is* the leading cause of death and disability among young people, making it an important public health problem. The dollar expenditure is staggering — some $25 billion yearly — and the costs in terms of human suffering are immeasurable.

Until brain injury occurs, most families pay it little attention. This book challenges us all to become involved and concerned. In an era that could bring fundamental reform to the health care system, and a human services bureaucracy that becomes more and more removed, it is important that we learn how to effectively navigate the system. It underscores the need for consumers to be informed, assertive, and stubbornly persistent in their quest for services in a system that has become top-heavy with red tape.

Filled with human drama, valuable information, and real life experiences, the book traces the steps of one family who fought their way through the system, survived, and learned to deal with the many challenges of living with a brain injured person. Along the way, it provides important insights into coping and advocacy. Patt Abrahamson is in a unique position to write this book because of her triangular role as a loving parent, caregiver, and trained social worker.

As the only national organization dedicated to the cause of brain injury, the Brain Injury Association supports the effort of all families who often must find their way alone. This book will help. Through the Family Resource Network, publications, as well as educational offerings, the Brain Injury Association is able to assist thousands of families every year. Through its Headsmart program and public policy advocacy, it is also active in promoting measures to prevent brain injuries, because prevention is the only known "cure." Another mission of the Brain Injury Association is to enhance the quality of life for people with a brain injury and their families, and this book will help the Brain Injury Association fulfill its mission.

Washington, D.C.

Forward by Former Congressman James Slattery (D-Kansas)
U.S. House of Representatives
Traumatic Brain Injury Act Sponsor

Brain Injury: A Family Tragedy is a hope-filled and gripping book depicting the drama of one family's attempt to deal with traumatic brain injury (TBI). The Abrahamson family's story is personally riveting and confirms and strengthens my support for the need for legislation dealing with brain injury. I first discovered the need for such legislation on May 20, 1993, when I received a letter from Jaclyn Anderson, an Independent Living Counselor at Three Rivers, Inc. Independent Living Resource Center, located in Wamego, Kansas. In her letter, she explained to me the trauma of brain injury for the survivor as well as their family, and she asked me to sponsor legislation, the Traumatic Brain Injury Act, that would assist victims of traumatic brain injury.

In human and economic terms, traumatic brain injury is one of the most devastating injuries a person can sustain. Those sustaining a severe brain injury typically face five to ten years of intensive medical and related services. It is estimated that $86,000 is needed per year for individuals to receive treatment for their brain injuries. This totals over $4 million in lifetime costs. With over 500,000 individuals who require hospitalization per year due to brain injuries, society incurs $25 billion per year in direct and indirect costs of medical treatment, rehabilitative and support services, and lost income. *Brain Injury: A Family Tragedy* illustrates this very real financial consequence, in addition to the wrenching emotional, mental, and physical consequences of brain injury.

Survivors of TBI are among the most under-served populations in our country, often receiving incorrect diagnoses and inappropriate treatment, and sometimes no treatment at all. Survivors of severe TBI are often inappropriately institutionalized solely in order to receive subsistence care. In addition, families of survivors of TBI often have no other choice but to institutionalize their loved ones in lieu of home- and community-based programs. *Brain Injury: A Family Tragedy* illustrates this very real trade-off.

I believe the Traumatic Brain Injury Act will provide states the opportunity to access federal funds that are necessary for expanding additional services statewide. The legislation will assist states in creating advisory boards to coordinate citizen participation in community traumatic brain injury programs, and will create a registry to advance epidemiological research efforts across the nation. This Act also calls for major studies to be conducted on the causes and prevention of brain injury. It also emphasizes the discovery and use of unique ways to prevent injury and heighten individual responsibility.

I am pleased that the State of Kansas was the first state to submit and receive approval on a Title XIX Home and Community Based Services Waiver to provide services to people with head injuries in their own home. I am hopeful that this legislation will encourage other States to develop home care programs for traumatic brain injury survivors and will create a nationwide network for survivors and their families and friends. The Traumatic Brain Injury Act, which emphasizes prevention and treatment options, will help these individuals and their families cope with the debilitating and lifelong consequences of these tragic accidents. *Brain Injury: A Family Tragedy* will help people understand the serious consequences of traumatic brain injury and the enormous challenges faced by traumatic brain injury survivors and their families. I am honored to have participated in a small way to help this book become a reality.

Washington, D.C.

Forward by Congressman Frank Pallone, Jr. (D-NJ)
U.S. House of Representatives
Traumatic Brain Injury Act Sponsor

Traumatic brain injury is a silent epidemic, quietly claiming its victims, many in the prime of their lives, without the sort of public alarm that would accompany an infectious disease outbreak of this magnitude. Another American will sustain a brain injury in the length of time it takes to read this paragraph. The numbers are staggering, yet the attention is scant.

Brain Injury: A Family Tragedy shares the arduous journey of a family caring for a traumatic brain injury victim. For those experiencing similar circumstances in caring for their loved one, it will prove an illustrative resource of another family's trials and tribulations; for other readers, it will open their eyes to the world of traumatic brain injury and prove educational. It is clear that a traumatic brain injury could strike any family.

While much more needs to be done, I am glad that I was able to play a part in the enactment of the Traumatic Brain Injury Act. As a co-author of this new law, it is my hope that there will be a greater focus on the plight of traumatic brain injury and its human, as well as economic, costs. It is a small investment that will have a large impact on research, effective diagnosis, prevention and education. More attention needs to be brought to this disability and I encourage every reader to become more involved with organizations like the national Brain Injury Association to help educate the public and advocate for more funding for research to benefit traumatic brain injury sufferers.

Washington, D.C.

Forward by John M. Porter, C.S.W.
Services Supervisor
Michigan Rehabilitation Services

Brain Injury: A Family Tragedy describes one family's travels through the maze of cognitive dysfunction. Whatever puzzlement the author's son experiences, it is equaled by that encountered by his loved ones in their interactions with physicians, psychologists and rehabilitation experts. Unlike Gary, they have the cognitive tools to make sense of the confusion.

The author displays an insight sharpened by the undergraduate social work education she began after the family was thrust into the world of traumatic brain injury. As much about her and her awakening as it is about her son, it describes the emerging role of self-advocate assumed by people with disabilities and by their family members. As an educated consumer and provider of social work services, she seems to have almost completed the transformation from a lifestyle of comfort and stability to one typified by continual challenge and chaos. How she has extracted attention and services from the medical establishment and from reluctant social agencies is a lesson worth learning. Too many consumers and their families are worn down and exhausted by others' efforts to deny them access to systems.

Patt has created systems where none existed. She has convinced service providers to begrudgingly authorize services which should have been offered freely. In writing of these challenges, she has shared her naiveté and her human frailty as well as her private thoughts and public victories.

While some may have seen her focus on Gary's improved functioning as a symptom of her own perseveration, many others will now see the triumph of a loving mother over the indifference and incompetency of those with greater knowledge and authority. Describing her own insights and inspirations, she spurs to action, with increased sensitivities, those of us in the helping professions who have not yet abandoned the idealism and hope with which we began our careers.

Marquette, MI

1

INITIAL TRAGEDY

May you live all the days of your life.
- Jonathan Swift

I slept later than usual that fateful Sunday. The details of that day, October 25, 1987, are still etched in my memory.

I woke up troubled by the recollection of a dream. As I sipped my coffee, I discussed the dream with my husband Gary Senior. "It seemed so real," I explained. "In my dream, we were boarding a plane when I realized I had forgotten to pack my shoes. I turned to tell you, and you collapsed before my eyes. I fell on top of you trying to perform CPR. Then I thought: *I don't know CPR! He's going to die because I've never had CPR training.* I was panicking. I felt helpless. I watched the life drain from your body."

"Do you suppose this could be a premonition?" I asked. I'm not usually superstitious, but my dream so took hold of me that I decided I should pursue CPR training. After all, Gary Senior *did* have open-heart surgery twelve years ago, and it was conceivable that this frightening dream could become reality.

That day paralleled our usual Sunday in October — having a leisurely breakfast, attending mass at St. Anne's Church, reading the Sunday paper, and (for my husband) watching the Green Bay Packers.

Our lives were serene and relaxed. Our three children were grown, married and living their own lives. We were at a pivotal point in our lives and felt we had earned the right to indulge ourselves. I didn't suffer from empty-nest syndrome as many women do. I had a life beyond child rearing and the home. We owned and operated a couple of dry-cleaning establishments. I had even secured a small business loan on my own to open a health club. The fitness challenge became a way of life for us. We ate, slept, and talked business and fitness. We awakened each morning eager to pursue new challenges.

Dining out that Sunday evening, the conversation reverted to my dream. Perhaps I was troubled by my husband's health problems. Life was so good for us. *Was that destined to change?* I worried that something might rob us of what we had together. I thought about his mortality, his vulnerability. *Am I a fatalist?*

We returned home about 8 p.m. I hit the play button on the answering machine and felt the blood drain from my head as I listened to an unfamiliar voice: "Call Kansas immediately. Your son has had a heart attack!"

I felt dizzy and faint. My husband stared in disbelief. *How can this be?* Gary Junior, our first born, was only 37 years old, an avid jogger in excellent health. Stunned, I contacted the hospital in Great Bend, Kansas. Gary and his family had lived in Great Bend the past five years. Kris, Gary's wife, seemed almost calm: "They are still working on Gary," she said. "He has had a cardiac arrest and is unconscious. He's alive and clinging to life," she continued, "but the prognosis looks dismal." Feelings of helplessness came over me at the realization that I was a thousand miles away from him.

I called throughout the night. The doctor's reports were chilling: "Still living ... unconscious ... not much hope ... virtually no chance of survival ... everything is against him." The doctor continued: "The cardiac arrest was complicated by a serious arrhythmia and inhaling vomit into the lungs. His chances of survival are almost nil." My mind reeled. *He's talking about my son!* Then, "Come immediately — the family needs support."

We live in Michigan's Upper Peninsula where, although the quality of life is unsurpassed, flights out of our area are limited. We left Escanaba at dawn after a traumatic exchange of phone calls to our other two children, Jeff in New York City and Vicki in Menominee, Michigan. We picked up Vicki en route to Milwaukee then flew to Wichita, where Jeff met us.

From there, a two-hour drive would bring us to Great Bend, Kansas, and to our son Gary.

The lack of sleep and tension left us physically and mentally exhausted. During the flight my thoughts wandered as I peered out the tiny window into miles of sky. I recalled the day Gary was born in Chicago. My husband and I were a couple of kids; I was 17 and Gary Senior was 19. Although I was young, I felt competent to care for my little son. After all, my mother started a second family when I was 12, and four more babies screamed their way into the world before I reached 16. I delighted in helping to care for them.

My first-born child! I was so proud of him. In the spring, he had received his associate's degree from Barton County Community College in Great Bend, Kansas. This was a milestone for Gary, who was typical of the flower child era in the late sixties, defiant of the establishment. His neat, short hair now made it difficult to remember the long, limp, straggly hair in which he delighted during high school. At last he had a direction and a goal. His recent letters were full of newfound pride: an A in both chemistry and microbiology. He was excited about his accomplishments. The future looked bright and promising. He was working to become a nurse anesthetist.

More memories came alive as we raced through the sky: my baby boy in a bassinet; the move to Sault Ste. Marie, Michigan when he was six; his quick little body running up and down the ice with a puck and a hockey stick; our move back to Escanaba, where he graduated from high school. Before this tragedy, I imagined our first trip to Kansas would be to attend his graduation from nursing school. Instead, we were racing the clock to see him alive one more time. Our precious boy!

Please, God, keep him alive until we arrive, I prayed. *Let me tell him one last time how much I love him.* Of course I loved him, but why hadn't I said it more often?

I remembered my dream, which was eerily similar to what was now taking place in my life. Like the dream, my husband and I had boarded a plane that morning, but it was my son (not my husband) who had collapsed; and it was his wife (not me) who had administered CPR. It was not an exact match;

still, I shivered at the uncanniness of it.

We arrived in Wichita at 7:00 p.m. on Monday. The two-hour drive seemed endless as we followed the narrow road to Great Bend. My first trip to Kansas: I expected to see amber waves of grain and breathe fresh country air. Instead, influenced by my mood, my senses focused more on the occasional smell of cow manure and the rhythmic movement of oil rigs dotting the countryside.

As we neared the city, my apprehension grew. The thought of seeing Gary suffer frightened me. I wept softly, felt my husband's comforting arm slip around me, and realized I wasn't alone in my grief.

The hospital came into view at last. We hurried into the lobby, found the elevator, then rushed down the long hall to the Intensive Care Unit. How frightening was that first glimpse. A sinking feeling came over me. The hissing and beeping of the cold steel machines keeping my son alive was terrifying. Monitors, tubes, and bottles of fluid were suspended everywhere. I gasped as I noticed the respirator. It hissed as it plunged up and down in synchrony with his swelling and deflating chest.

His blue eyes were large and frightened. Sweat poured down his face. His eyes filled with tears as his Adam's apple moved downward trying to swallow, as if he were engulfed by grief and pain. Although he couldn't speak, I felt he was aware of my presence.

"Gary, I love you so," I whispered in his ear.

The doctor looked haggard as he motioned us into the hall. Again, he explained the gravity of our son's condition.

"Gary is having irregular heart beats," he said. "Even if the heart stabilizes, the lungs are badly compromised. He has adult respiratory distress syndrome caused from aspirating vomit into the lungs." Apparently, it is not unusual for a heart failure victim to vomit, and then swallow some of it while gasping for air.

"The chances of survival are remote," the doctor explained. "If he does survive, he has been without oxygen to the brain; there is almost certain to be brain damage — possibly severe."

We cried, prayed together, and hugged one another in an effort at consolation. Guilt, anger, denial, anguish, humility, and bitterness — yes, I felt them all, but I clung to my faith and never stopped praying.

The next couple of days were a nightmare as Gary's condition regressed. Lung shock set in, as the doctor had predicted. Trying to fight off the foreign particles, his lungs filled with fluid. A pulmonary specialist from Wichita was consulted.

"We must perform a bronchoscopy," he declared. "It is all there is left. Hopefully, the procedure will buy some time, and if we have to do it three, four, or even ten times, we will."

I became nauseated as he described the procedure. The bronchoscope is introduced into the throat, past the vocal cords into the trachea, and down into the bronchial tubes, causing suffocation during the procedure. Kris signed the necessary papers and we retreated to the chapel, where we prayed together.

Twelve hours later, at 5:00 a.m. on Thursday, the hospital told us Gary's lungs were again filling up and the bronchoscopy would have to be repeated. It was raining, dreary, and dark as we rushed back to the hospital.

"Gary seems to be compensating on his own now," the doctor explained solemnly, "but I am going ahead with the procedure as planned." A small piece of emesis, or vomit, was again extracted from the lungs.

We visited the small, unpretentious chapel on the hospital grounds often. The strength we needed was not to be found in our secular world.

In the chapel, a young man approached us: "I'm Mitch Webster, a friend of your son's," he said. "We go to the same church." Mitch Webster was one of fifty or so members of the community that offered support and consolation to Gary's family. Mitch had heard of the tragedy at church. My husband, a sports buff, knew him instantly as a professional baseball player for Montreal. As Mitch joined us in a circle of prayer, I was struck by the level and intensity of support displayed by so many in the community. The small waiting room near the intensive care unit was always filled with friends from the Baptist church where Gary and Kris were members. They prayed, consoled us, and brought food to Gary's home.

The next day, the lungs appeared to stabilize; periodic suctioning was administered to prevent fluid build-up in the lungs. As Gary became more lucid, a nurse reported that she communicated with Gary by having him blink his eyes. Meanwhile, Gary began to fight the respirator to breathe on his own. Then, the doctor announced he was going to try some aggressive therapy. He turned the respirator down, requiring Gary to use more of his own impaired resources to breathe, and left the room for a phone call.

Suddenly, something was wrong! I sensed it. Gary's eyes bulged out as if to, hysterically, plead for help. It was clear that he needed the machine and was not yet ready to be weaned from it. His wife looked on apprehensively as the room filled with nurses and the respiratory therapy supervisor arrived. Apparently, as Gary struggled for air, he managed to dislodge the respirator tube that had been placed in his throat to feed him oxygen. Gary lapsed into a coma. His first seizure took place a few hours later.

Endless hours passed while we waited for a sign of life. Kris talked of that Sunday, reliving the dreadful moments. "Gary was stretching out after his usual five-mile jog," she explained, "when suddenly the dogs started to bark violently. They never bark, so I ran to the doorway to see what the commotion was. I heard an agonizing groan that seemed almost animal-like. I saw Gary on the grass, collapsed; the dogs were barking frantically over his body, as if they sensed what was happening. In seconds, I was over him, performing CPR, stopping long enough to scream, 'Arlo, call an ambulance! Your dad is unconscious!' They arrived almost instantly since the hospital is only two blocks away. That's probably one reason Gary survived. The paddles were positioned on Gary's chest. One jolt — nothing. Two more jolts. His limp body would spring from the ground with each jolt. 'We've got a beat,' one medic said. 'Let's get him to the hospital.'"

"Suddenly, I was aware of being barefoot," Kris continued. "I hesitated; should I go in the house for my shoes or go without them? Someone helped me into the ambulance. Suddenly, Gary vomited. Vomit flew into the air, onto the medic, and into both of their eyes. The apparatus used to suction the lungs didn't work. Gary's heart stopped again as we reached the hospital."

As Kris told her story, I shuddered at the missing shoes in my dream; the dream now seemed like less of a mere coincidence and more like a foggy premonition of our future.

Both of Gary's sons had also witnessed the medics working on their dad. The oldest, Arlo, was 14 at the time of the incident; Leif Eric was eight. My brother-in-law Glenn, Gary's favorite uncle, and his wife Alexis came from Colorado as soon as they heard about Gary. They cared for the boys while Kris kept vigil at Gary's bedside.

Gary Senior and I were concerned about Gary being in a small hospital. We urged Kris to move him to a major medical center. There was no pulmonologist on staff at Great Bend, and we naturally wanted to give Gary every advantage. Kris was, at first, reluctant because the nearest large facility was two hours away in Wichita — away from home, away from the support group. Moreover, what if his lungs should fill again during the airlift?

Soon, we were faced with a decision point. On Friday afternoon, shortly after Gary's first seizure, the doctor held a family conference. He told us that Gary's heart was beginning to fail. We discussed the idea of a move with the doctor. He initially responded that not much more could be done — that they were doing all they could.

Not entirely satisfied with this response, I asked:

"Doctor, what would *you* do if this was *your* son?"

He paused, momentarily stared ahead, and then yielded.

"I guess I would want the best medical treatment available."

2

SURVIVAL

One can survive anything these days except death.
- Oscar Wilde

Still comatose, Gary was transferred via air ambulance to St. Francis Hospital in Wichita. One week had passed since the initial tragedy.

St. Francis was built around a small chapel that dated back to 1889. Gary Senior and I attended mass their twice daily. Not that we were overly religious: in fact, there had been times in past years that we attended church only infrequently. However, during this time of uncertainty, chaos, and grief, that chapel nourished us like food, giving us needed strength.

At the hospital, a pulmonary specialist and a neurologist were consulted. Several tests were run to evaluate Gary's condition. He continued to baffle doctors by clinging to life.

The neurologist, a small beady-eyed man who looked almost sinister, approached my husband and me with a solemn look: "Gary is in a vegetative state," he said. "He has brain stem damage, seizures, and no cranial response. Death is imminent."

I ran down the hall, blocking my ears with my hands. *He's wrong! My son can't die; this isn't happening!*

My husband, more controlled than I, questioned the doctor more thoroughly: "How long *will* he live in this state?"

"Not more than three weeks," the doctor impassively replied. "His vital organs will fail, causing death."

The days that followed were agonizing. Kris, Gary Senior, and I alternated the vigil by Gary's bedside. Monitors frightened me as I watched his heart rate rise and fluctuate wildly during a seizure. His blood pressure would reach 200 over 110. His arms would flail in the air as if he were a puppet attached to invisible strings. I worried that he might be in pain. Nurses suctioned his lungs regularly. His temperature was out of control as sweat poured from his face and body. I wiped his forehead and continuously talked to him. Occasionally, his eyes would flutter. "Reflexes," the nurses explained, dashing my hopes. "Not purposeful."

One day his arms and legs turned inward and stiffened. "Look, he can move," I said, thinking this was a good sign. "The movement is decorticate and decerebrate posturing — a primitive response to pain," a nurse explained. "Primitive reflexes."

Kris was the first to notice gross movements. His arms raised as if trying to grab the endotracheal tube. To avoid pulling out the tube accidently, she asked that his arms be softly restrained, particularly when family members were not around to observe.

Then there came a change. Gary began to blink on command and to track the movements of people in the room with his eyes. I rejoiced, like a mother observing her child's first step.

After days of begging Gary to squeeze my hand, I felt the first faint squeeze. Not trusting my judgment, I asked my husband to place his hand in Gary's. He felt the squeeze also! We ran to get a nurse. Gary did not squeeze her hand when she asked him to. "Non-purposeful reflexes," she soberly asserted.

The doctor came in the room for his daily visit. He stood stiffly in the doorway with his arms folded. I exclaimed our new-found revelation: "Gary squeezed my hand! Please, come over here and see!" He made no attempt to alter his stance or to accommodate my request. Frustrated by the doctor's aloofness, Gary Senior broke the silence: "Can't you even give her the courtesy of letting her show you his hand squeeze? Don't you have any humanity in you? Gary's mother sees some small ray of hope and you refuse to acknowledge it. What are you made of, anyway?"

At this, my concern turned to my husband. Two years before, he had a stroke; there was no residual effect, but I worried about the threat to him posed by all the stress. The next time I saw the doctor, he advised me to get psychiatric help for my husband. He also stated that if there were any further outbursts, he would leave orders barring us from visiting Gary.

I realize now that their negative outlook and guarded responses were partly an attempt to discourage what may turn out to be false hopes. Nevertheless, it was difficult to deal with the absolute pessimism of the hospital staff. We found out later that the victim may respond mainly to family members as the coma first lifts.

Though paralyzed, Gary continued to become more alert. About five weeks after his cardiac arrest, Gary was taken off of the respirator. Without this obstruction in Gary's throat area, verbal communication was possible. Although at first he seemed fairly normal — appropriately answering "yes" or "no" to simple questions — it soon became clear that his brain function was anything but normal. For example, if I would leave his room for an hour or so, upon returning he would comment: "Mom, how are you? I haven't seen you in years."

Physically, things weren't much better. His weight had fallen from a pre-cardiac arrest 160 pounds to only 132 pounds. He had to relearn simple things like swallowing; until he could swallow on his own, he received nourishment through a feeding tube inserted through his nose down toward his stomach area. He was also paralyzed from the waist down, making him incontinent — both bladder and bowel.

Soon, however, he stabilized enough to be moved out of the critical care unit to another floor. Kris and I took turns sleeping on a cot in his room. One of the daily drugs he took helped control the frequency and duration of his seizures.

Then, in what seemed to be a major setback, Gary stiffened, becoming almost comatose. The staff rushed to do tests. I felt my hope for Gary's survival drain. I went to the lobby and called my husband. I couldn't stop crying. But when I returned to Gary's room, the problem was alleviated. Apparently, he had coughed up the feeding tube, which had coiled up in his throat, compromising his breathing.

This was the second such incident with the feeding tube. Earlier, Kris had witnessed thick blue fluid bubbling out of his mouth. The tube had dislodged from the stomach and he aspirated (accidently inhaling food into his lungs), causing an aspiration pneumonia.

We were on an emotional roller coaster, up one day, down the next. Our moods moved in synchrony to changes in Gary's condition.

Kris, Gary Senior, and I stayed at a motel two blocks from the hospital. Kris spent nights at the hospital with Gary; Gary Senior and I were with him during the day.

One night at the motel, I felt like I couldn't breathe. Terrified, I awakened my husband as I struggled for oxygen. We rushed to the emergency room. I was positive I was dying. Although concerned about my son on the second floor, I forced the thought of him from my mind. I had to be concerned with *my* survival now!

After an examination, a shot, and prescription medicine, I was reassured that my episode was stress-related.

As time passed, Gary Senior decided to return home to Michigan. We had left in a state of fear and confusion. Someone had to look into the operations of our business.

Kris returned to her job in Great Bend. On weekends, she came to be with Gary. Sometimes, the minister and members of their church would also come. On one occasion, we formed a powerful prayer circle at Gary's bedside. His eyes were open, but he looked bewildered and confused.

I bought Gary a balloon and attached it to his bed. Like a child, he would bat at the balloon.

From his room, you could see the elevator, with its constant stream of people coming and going. Their figures reflected off the window in his room. Gary would point to the window and appear anxious and frightened, thinking people were coming through the window. I could not reason with him about this.

He was on the fourth floor. While he slept, I sat and gazed out his window. On more than one occasion, I watched the life-lift helicopter land, rushing a person in distress into the elevator door on the roof. I empathized with the traumatized person as well as the family; chances are, they had little insight into the months of distress that could lay ahead.

One evening, Kris and I sat in the lounge while Gary received treatment to strengthen his breathing. Kris began to reflect on their marriage. The first years were difficult. Gary floated from job to job. His dissatisfaction with entry-level jobs stemmed from his perception that he was capable of much more.

Kris revealed a possible drinking problem of which I was unaware. "He was a binge-type drinker," she explained, "not drinking for weeks at a time. I gave him an ultimatum: shape up or else! For the past five years, it hasn't been a problem. We have a wonderful relationship. Gary is a great father to the boys. Finally, our life is on track. Gary's doing well in school. We attend church as a family. It couldn't be better. Now this tragedy. It isn't fair."

Kris was an occupational therapy instructor at the college, and Gary had taken the job of school photographer to help finance his own schooling. He had earned the respect of professionals and peers alike.

I sympathized with Kris and offered my own recollections. Gary's early years were spent in Sault Ste. Marie, Michigan. Hockey and skating dominated our existence. As a hockey player, Gary experienced great success. We followed his all-star team to Canada and international tournaments. Gordy Howe was his idol. In 1966, we moved back to Escanaba — the town in which Gary Senior and I grew up — when Gary was a sophomore.

Essentially, Gary was a good boy, always honest. But he had a certain naiveté about him and sometimes exhibited a tendency to be more a follower than a leader. On occasion, he displayed bad judgment. For example, during his junior year, he was on the football team. Friday night was to be parents' night. Gary Senior and I were looking forward to attending the game. Unfortunately, things didn't turn out the way we expected. Without provocation, Gary ran away with another boy who was experiencing growing pains and problems at home. For six weeks, we didn't know where he was or whether he was even alive. They turned up in New Orleans. Gary called and wanted to come home. He said he knew he had made a mistake the first night he left home, while sleeping on the side of the road, cold and hungry.

We talked about the Zeitgeist of the times — the 60's: long hair, rebellion, and marijuana. Gary was influenced by these factors. Nevertheless, Gary was very popular with his peers, considered a neat dresser and a good dancer. The girls thought he was extremely handsome. He was probably not too different from a majority of young people at that time.

I recalled a special time in 1985, two years before his cardiac arrest. Gary's younger brother Jeff, who worked in a congressional office in Washington, D.C., announced his forthcoming wedding. Gary was in the wedding party. The occasion stands out in my mind because a new side of the many-faceted Gary was unfolding. I was especially proud of the maturity he displayed. Gary had turned the corner, and it showed. He displayed both sensitivity and assertiveness. At the wedding, he seemed to take charge as he ushered me down the aisle of St. Peter's Cathedral near Capitol Hill. It was a posh wedding with an elegant reception at the Fort Myers Officers Club in Arlington, Virginia. In attendance were members of Congress and many staffers from Capitol Hill. Gary knew protocol. He fit in now, and he knew it.

Kris went back into Gary's room. I retreated to the cafeteria to give them time alone. My mind was swirling with our conversation as I reflected on the sometimes turbulent relationship my husband and I had with Kris.

My first recollection of Kris was in 1971, during a visit she made to our dry cleaning business, located in a shopping mall. Our daughter Vicki and Kris came in while we were working one evening. I was waiting on a customer in the lobby as I caught a glimpse of her. She was extremely tall — close to six feet — and very thin. She was wearing blue jeans and a short, cropped jacket. As I looked at her from my own height of 5'2", it seemed that her legs dominated her form. Her face was thin, with white-blonde hair hanging out of a large black hat with a floppy brim and a tall, u-shaped crown. I was engaged in conversation with the customer and did not

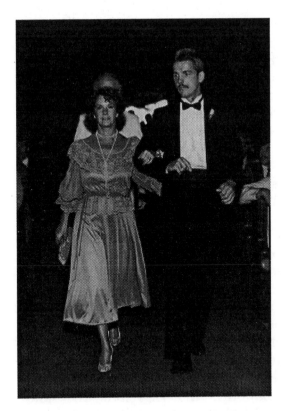

Gary escorts his mom down
the aisle at his brother Jeff's
wedding, 1985.

speak to Kris at that time.

At home that evening, I questioned Vicki: "Who was that girl with you? I've never seen her before..." "Oh, that was Kris Ostlund," she replied. I commented on her unconventional, hippie-like appearance. Actually, she was probably considered very hip by her peers. Vicki responded, "Well, get used to it; your son is dating her!"

The next time we saw Kris, Gary introduced us formally. Gary invited her to join us in attending my younger sister's wedding. She sat in the back seat of the car, speaking mainly to Gary about some cookies she had made. While her inattentiveness toward Gary Senior and I could have been mistaken for unfriendly behavior, it was probably mere shyness.

The next thing I knew, they were living together on the outskirts of town with three of Gary's friends. Two months later, Gary announced they were going to marry. Kris' parents wanted a sedate wedding, only a few family members at a restaurant. Gary and Kris, who were only a few years beyond high school, wanted a larger wedding for the family as well as their many friends. We rented a hall for them. About 150 young people attended their reception. The restauranteur commented on the well-behaved polite, young people in attendance.

For their wedding, Gary chose a grey-black tuxedo with tails and a top hat. Kris made her own wedding dress out of a pink and lilac flower print on a cream background. They were married in a small, unpretentious church outside of town. There was a stream of red carpet running down the aisle. The minister was a hippie friend of theirs. The wedding was supposed to be held in a field, but the weather didn't cooperate.

The church filled with young people. Friends recited poems, played guitars, and sang beautiful ballads. It turned out to be a most beautiful wedding as Gary and Kris exchanged vows and began their life together.

From the point of view of our conservative generation, we thought they were peculiar. Kris' mother related the same feelings. Jokingly, she wondered whether they mixed up the babies in the hospital where she had delivered Kris. Surely, this must be someone else's child!

I entered the elevator to return to Gary's room. Despite our differences over the years, this tragedy had ironically brought Kris and me closer than ever — a potential silver lining in an otherwise very unhappy situation.

Gary was sitting up in a chair when I returned. He wanted to get back in bed. Because he was still paralyzed from the waist down, Kris and I attempted to move him ourselves. He was dead weight, and we nearly dropped him. Finally, all three of us fell on the bed together, with Gary in the middle. Gary looked baffled and bewildered while Kris and I laughed hysterically. I ran to the bathroom, unable to hold my water, still laughing uncontrollably. The nurse came in to see what the commotion was. Kris laughed as she joked, "That's just my mother-in-law having a fit." Yes, we had developed a close-

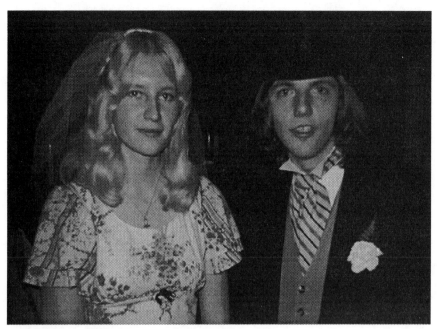

Gary and Kris on their wedding day, 1972.

ness. I believed we saw in one another things we wouldn't let ourselves see before then.

Thanksgiving was spent at the Ronald McDonald House, where eventually we were able to get a room. Everyone there was very hospitable and seemed genuinely concerned for each other. Finally, we weren't alone in our tragedy. I don't have enough accolades for the Ronald McDonald House. It was a home away from home. On one occasion, Gary's tape player was stolen from the hospital and the Ronald McDonald staff replaced it for him.

Two months had passed since Gary's cardiac arrest. His condition stabilized. The medical staff felt that Gary would benefit from intense physical and cognitive therapies at another Wichita institution more adept at rehabilitation, St. Joseph's Medical Center.

As we waited in Gary's room to depart to St. Joseph's, I sensed a combination of excitement and relief in Gary. "I can't wait to get out of this hell hole," he exclaimed.

I observed how handsome Gary appeared in his electric

blue sweat suit that deepened the blue in his eyes. This was the first occasion in more than two months that Gary was able to wear street clothes.

I can only imagine the thoughts that might have reverberated in his brain injured head. In an attempt to place blame on someone, something, or someplace for the confusion he was experiencing, perhaps he blamed this "hell hole." Surely leaving it would correct the injustices imposed upon him. Maybe life would begin to make sense again. One seemingly lucid moment a few days earlier, he begged: "Get me out of here, Mom, before I lose my mind completely!"

The Kansas sky was blue, bright, and sunny on that first day of December, unlike the dismal, gray cloud cover that often blankets the Lake Michigan area at that time of year. New optimism surged as the ambulance sped across town to the rehabilitation center.

Gary had already beaten the odds. He had survived!

3

REHABILITATION

What cannot be cured must be endured.
- Francois Rabelais

Survival is instinctive. Faced with danger, we go to great lengths to assure the survival of ourselves or our loved ones. Mothers have been known to lift a car after an accident to free a pinned child.

Gary's situation was not that simple. There was no car for me to lift that would free Gary of his condition; if there were, adrenaline would have rushed through my veins, allowing me to do it.

But we did much more than sit by and hope for the best. We were able to be there for Gary, to pray, and to make sure that he was getting the best possible professional care. That combined with Gary's strong will to survive allowed him to elude dire predictions of imminent death.

Early on the doctors had warned us that *if* he survived, oxygen deprivation would almost certainly result in severe brain damage. Yet, the day-to-day survival mode of the first couple of months did not allow us to fully contemplate — much less prepare for — what lay ahead.

I had now entered the alien world of brain injury — an environment comparable to Bedlam, the famous, now defunct insane asylum in London. While medical technology helped rescue Gary from the throes of death, it failed to bring back the same person.

In the end, Gary could fully recover physically, but not mentally; the same technology that saves lives creates in its wake a whole new disability group. This sad fact became increasingly clear as we transitioned from survival mode to rehabilitation mode.

Upon arrival at St. Joseph's, we were escorted to a room half the size of Gary's previous one. He would share that room with a judge who recently had a stroke.

The admitting nurse garnered information with the usual questions. Gary seemed to take command as he answered historical questions about himself. Then the nurse asked, "Why are you here?" Gary replied, "to have my throat checked out (it was still sore from the respirator insult) and whatever it says on the paper," motioning to the paper in her hand. "Can't you read?" he asked sarcastically, in an effort to conceal his lack of understanding as to why he was there.

The nurse left the room. I turned my attention to the judge in the next bed, and to his wife. I introduced myself and Gary. In an attempt to be sociable, Gary asked the judge, "When did *you* arrive at this luxury hotel?" I momentarily pondered whether his inquiry stemmed from cynicism or a failure to understand the circumstances that had brought him here. The judge, a portly man, and obviously in a state of confusion due to his stroke, looked pleadingly to his wife for answers.

The remainder of the day proved rather routine until late afternoon, when the judge turned on the TV. Moments later, the judge began to sob and cry. His cries became louder. His wife, sensing my concern and puzzlement, explained that he was emotionally labile. He would laugh or cry uncontrollably, unable to put on the brakes. Gary squirmed. Appearing anxious and agitated, he began to shake and speak loudly. I buzzed for the nurse.

She arrived and immediately sensed the problem. A combination of a new environment, the confusion of a roommate crying, and the blaring television all set the stage for an accelerated event. We helped Gary into his wheelchair and proceeded into the hallway, attempting to liberate him from the confusion. His anxiety continued to escalate. He pounded on the wall with his head and hands, begging for help. "The world is coming to an end. We're all going to die! Do something! *Do something*, please, Mom," he pleaded.

Gary was given a sedative. When he quieted down, the

nurse explained that Gary was not only reacting to external events but to his own internal confusion as well. I returned to the Ronald McDonald house that evening unable to sleep. I waited for daylight.

Early the next morning, I talked with a social worker and the program director at the center. They advised me that they were going to get Gary a private room, with a special mattress to put on the floor. Gary would not — could not — be surrounded by noise and people. The mattress would also obviate the need to tie him in bed for safety purposes.

The following day, the mattressed room was ready. Gary fell into the mattress exclaiming, "Back to the real world," as he rolled back and forth, exerting his new-found freedom.

Kris and Leif came on the weekend. It was their first visit to the new hospital. They were pleased with the mattress arrangement. Leif jumped on the mattress and snuggled up to his dad as he always had in the past. Gary was close to Leif and called him "Peanut," but the conversation differed now. "Dad, do you know where you are? What day is it, Dad? Do you know what year it is?" I left the room to allow Kris, Gary, and Leif some time alone together.

Gary vacillated from being lucid and aware to confused and agitated in the days that followed. One day, when I entered his room, a nurse had apparently been stern with him in an attempt to get him to do something. Upon seeing me, he turned to the nurse and said, "Sure, go ahead and try to act nice to me in front of my mother, you hypocrite!" He was so convincing, I wondered if he did have some memory of mistreatment. I'll never know.

Gary exhibited bouts of paranoid behavior. He was convinced that staff members at the center were trying to poison him. He refused medication. He was much more cooperative when either Kris or I were there to orient him to place and time and explain what had happened to him.

As I reflect on those incidents now, I believe his reaction — at least on some level — may actually have been logical. I can only speculate about what Gary's perspective might have been. But, imagine you're in a strange place, not knowing how or when you got there, tied to a bed at night and a wheel-chair during the day, not able to separate dream from reality, and totally confused by a lack of moment-to-moment memory. Naturally he thought *they* were the enemy. Of course he thought *they* were trying to poison him. In a remote, rational corner of his brain, he thought the pills must be the culprit: *they*, the staff, the institution, were altering his mind! *Why?*

Gary always knew family members. On many occasions when I walked into his room, he chided me for not visiting him. "I haven't seen you in five years," he would lament. Sometimes, I had only left the room to go to the cafeteria. In any case, Gary's behavior was calmer, and usually more appropriate, when a family member was with him, or when a family member telephoned him.

His skin had broken down from his lack of bladder control. The staff took care to avert more skin breakdown. An external catheter was placed in his penis with a line tied to a bag on his leg. Hanging from his leg like a huge balloon, the urine-filled bag was repulsive. "Get this off me!" he once screamed. He would tug at his leg and wail about an operation he had. One day he told me, "Have someone check out my balls; something's wrong with them — they're humongous!"

Carl (not his real name) was a male nurse assigned to Gary. In Gary's paranoid mind, Carl wore a black hat. The director of the facility explained that brain injured patients oftentimes view staff members as either wearing black hats or white hats, like the good and bad cowboys in old Westerns.

I noted the agitation that ensued whenever Carl came into the room. Reviewing the nursing notes, I discovered that Gary had threatened to kill Carl. Whenever Carl was around, Gary went on the offensive — verbally and sometimes physically. He tried to grab Carl whenever he came within reach. More than one entry said that Gary "struck staff with call light."

I also noted that medication to calm Gary was almost always administered when Carl was assigned to Gary. On several occasions, Carl had other staff members help hold Gary down for 20 to 30 minutes until a shot took hold.

I chide myself now for not being more assertive about all this. I should have insisted that Carl not be assigned to Gary.

At the time, I sensed a lack of compassion and sensitivity in Carl. I tried to dismiss those thoughts, as if they were a figment of my imagination.

My perception of medical professionals, especially doctors, was that they are near infallible. Years ago, few questioned the wisdom of these professionals; whatever they said was gospel. Today, I question that "wisdom." As you march through life, experiences make you much more assertive.

I learned that when a loved one is in the hospital, family members and others can play an important role — as advocate, overseer, and guardian. To assure the best possible care, you have to take responsibility for your loved one. Mistakes are frequently made, oversights occur. To a nurse or a doctor, your loved one is just one of many patients. Don't place your total trust in the facility. Be the eyes and ears for the medical staff when they're not around. Ask questions, anticipate, be both assertive and observant.

As the days passed, a new brain injury language, completely foreign to me, began to unravel. For example, a brain injured person, whose injury prevents him from understanding something, will often "confabulate" — construct a plausible story to explain it. With Gary, confabulation was rampant. On one occasion, he complained to a nurse that he had been beaten then robbed; he warned that suspicious cars were outside his room. Later, he tearfully told the nurses, "my father has died."

One evening, I cleaned his nose with cotton swabs. The next morning, he confabulated that he had an operation on his nose. He told me in great detail how they had put huge tubes up his nostrils. Everything was exaggerated. He confabulated about operations on his brain, his throat, and his testicles.

One afternoon, I heard a baby crying across the hall. I was told the cries were that of a two-year-old girl with a brain injury. That evening, Gary lifted his sheets and told me there were three babies lying by his feet. He insisted that I remove them. He said they wouldn't stop crying.

As he progressed physically, he was able to get around the floor in his wheelchair. One day, I couldn't find Gary.

After a search, we found him in someone else's room drinking everything in sight. One day, he parked at the nursing station and drank out of a huge, heavy pitcher, spilling water everywhere.

The roller coaster continued. Gary became sick. He moaned and vomited. Blood tests showed that the medication he took to control seizures had reached toxic levels. At times, he appeared grossly over medicated, unresponsive, and lethargic. Sometimes his breathing would become shallow.

On good days he would participate in speech, occupational, and physical therapy. On some occasions, he was surprisingly appropriate; he once demanded to see his individual treatment plan. Overall, however, the drugs definitely limited his abilities.

The medical staff explained that after the coma lifts, a person progresses through various cognitive functioning stages. Medical and rehabilitative professionals sometimes use the Rancho Los Amigos Scale to describe these stages. Neither the ultimate outcome nor the pace of improvement can be accurately predicted, although most improvement usually takes place within the first two years. Gary could stop at any stage and not improve any further.

Physically, Gary made substantial progress. He relearned how to walk — almost robot-like, with a wide gait, but he *could* ambulate. His speech seemed intact, although his voice was still low from the respirator insult. He did substitute words, for example "branch" for "straw." The analogies were almost funny. Because of the rapid physical improvement, I assumed that meaningful cognitive improvement was just around the corner.

I even assumed that, in the future, Gary might be able to continue his schooling. Perhaps I wasn't prepared to accept a dismal prognosis at that point. I reasoned that the medical profession had been wrong in the past; hence, when they were now unable to provide me with concrete predictions about his future progress, I filled in the information gaps with best-case scenarios. Unwittingly, I may have been simply protecting myself. I wasn't yet ready to face reality.

As Christmas drew near, I realized I had to return to Michi-

RANCHO LOS AMIGOS SCALE

Levels of Cognitive Functioning

The Rancho Levels, as they are called, describe the various behavioral stages a brain injury victim may experience as he progresses through rehabilitation. Assessments are determined by observing the patient's response to environmental stimuli. An individual may plateau at any stage.

I **NO RESPONSE**: Patient appears to be in a deep sleep and is unresponsive to stimuli.

II **GENERALIZED RESPONSE**: Patient reacts inconsistently and non-purposefully to stimuli in a non-specific manner. Responses are limited and often the same, regardless of stimuli presented.

III **LOCALIZED RESPONSE**: Patient responses are specific but inconsistent, and are directly related to the type of stimulus presented, such as turning head toward a sound or focusing on a presented object. He may follow simple commands in an inconsistent and delayed manner.

IV **CONFUSED - AGITATED**: Patient is in a heightened state of activity and severely confused, disoriented, and unaware of present events. His behavior is frequently bizarre and inappropriate to his immediate environment. He is unable to perform self care. If not physically disabled, he may perform automatic motor activities such as sitting, reaching, and walking as part of his agitated state, but not necessarily as a purposeful act.

V **CONFUSED - INAPPROPRIATE, NON-AGITATED**: Patient appears alert and responds to simple commands. More complex commands, however, produce responses that are non-purposeful and random. The patient may show some agitated behavior triggered by external stimuli rather than internal confusion. The patient is highly distractible and generally has difficulty in learning new information. He can manage self-care activities with assistance. His memory is impaired and verbalization is often inappropriate.

VI **CONFUSED - APPROPRIATE**: Patient shows goal-directed behavior, but relies on cuing for direction. He can relearn old skills such as activities of daily living, but memory problems interfere with new learning. He has a beginning awareness of self and others.

VII **AUTOMATIC APPROPRIATE**: Patient goes through daily routine automatically, but is robot-like with appropriate behavior and minimal confusion. He has shallow recall of activities, and superficial awareness of, but lack of insight into, his condition. He requires at least minimal supervision because judgment, problem-solving, and planning skills are impaired.

VIII **PURPOSEFUL APPROPRIATE**: Patient is alert and oriented, and is able to recall and integrate past and present events. He can learn new activities and continue without supervision once the activities are learned. He is independent in home and living skills, though deficits in stress tolerance, judgment, abstract reasoning, social, emotional, and intellectual capacities may persist.

gan. My husband had left weeks earlier.

When I finally did return home, I couldn't eat, sleep, or think of anything but Gary. I called the rehabilitation center endlessly, sometimes three or four times a day. Gary never remembered the previous call, even if it had been just minutes before. At times he was so drugged, his speech was slurred and slow. Sometimes he fell asleep during the conversation. I would call the nursing station often for updates on his progress.

Kris was able to spend more time with Gary during Christmas vacation. She attended therapies with Gary. His strength increased as he ambulated with assistance.

One day, Kris called, extremely upset. She had returned home overnight to check on the boys and to get fresh clothes. In her absence, Gary had fallen out of the wheelchair, requiring several stitches above his eyebrow. She expressed concern about Gary being over medicated. After the fall, he again became unresponsive, according to nursing notes.

Kris and I talked again. "I'm worried about what will happen to Gary when school resumes and I have to go back to work," Kris said. "He doesn't do well without family here."

The rehabilitation center informed Kris that Gary would need 24-hour care when he was discharged, and that she should start looking into care arrangements or alternatives. They also told her to apply for Social Security Disability Income (SSDI) for Gary. The rehabilitation center also felt that Gary's chances of progress would be greater if family members could be present for a greater percentage of time.

I investigated the brain injury program in Marquette, Michigan, 65 miles from our home. It's the only program available in the Upper Peninsula where we live.

We reached a family consensus. Gary would be transported via air ambulance to Marquette for continued therapy. My husband and I would alternate staying at the hospital with Gary. Kris would finish the school year in Kansas. Subsequently, she and the boys would move back to Michigan.

Kris set into motion the paperwork required for the transfer. This was a difficult decision for Kris.

With a combination of sadness and optimism, Kris and Leif waved good-bye as they watched Gary's plane disappear into the horizon.

4

RETURN TO MICHIGAN

There is no greater sorrow than
to recall a happy time in the midst of sorrow.
- Dante

Seventy-six days after his cardiac arrest, on January 9, 1988, Gary arrived in Marquette via air ambulance. Gary Senior and I waited anxiously at the hospital for his arrival. A stretcher on wheels approached us, pushed by two orderlies.

"Hi, Mom. Hi, Dad," Gary greeted us with a smile on his shrunken face, seemingly unaware of his surroundings or why he was there. He raised his body on his elbows as they whisked him passed us.

It was about 8:00 p.m. We spent a couple of hours with Gary while a steady stream of nurses began the usual admitting procedures. The last time his father had seen him, Gary was still semicomatose and on a respirator. Gary Senior was startled and impressed with the progress he observed. We retreated to a nearby motel, chatting excitedly about our renewed optimism for Gary's recovery.

It didn't take long, however, to realize that Gary's bizarre behavior was still evident. Due in part to the loss of short-term memory and the resulting confusion, he was still paranoid.

He would look out the eighth floor window of Marquette General Hospital Regional Medical Center, view Sugar Loaf Mountain covered with snow in all its splendor, and swear he was in Colorado (he had lived there at one time). Some mornings he would look out the window and claim the streets and houses had been moved overnight.

He begged his father to report the inconsistencies to the police. It was impossible to reason with him. Then, in his frustration, he turned on his father, accusing him of "not being a man" because he wouldn't call the police. He taunted his father relentlessly. Gary Senior, thrown into the alien world of brain injury, finally buckled. Attempting to defend himself against Gary's steady attacks, he shot back, "I'm more of a man than you'll ever be," and left the room. Gary then stalked the halls, hunting for his father.

In his unit, Gary was the only brain injured person amongst many elderly stroke patients. As such, he tended to create quite a disturbance. Sometimes, to explain his bizarre behavior, Gary would confabulate. He told the therapists he was tired, that he'd been working all night, or had just returned from Chicago.

Speech, occupational, and physical therapy occupied daytime hours, but we soon found that these activities left Gary exhausted and agitated most of the time.

When the nurses picked up soiled clothing — which they did every day — Gary imagined that he was being "ripped off." He constantly opened and closed drawers, rearranging the contents, hiding things. On one occasion, he was changing his underpants (incontinence was a problem), and a ten dollar bill fell onto the floor. Apparently he had taken the money from my purse, possibly with the idea of helping him escape.

Sometimes, he stumbled shakily down the hall pounding on walls. He thought he was in prison but didn't know why. He confronted his father, threatening to kill him for causing whatever it was that had happened to him. He was like a little boy looking for someone to blame — some explanation to make sense of it all.

One evening, very late, one of the nurses called to asked if I would come help quiet Gary. As I entered the room, he had his underpants down, screaming that his "privates" were normal now. "Get a camera and take a picture," he pleaded. I wanted to laugh and cry at the same time.

The doctor gave us permission to take him home over the weekend. With some assistance, Gary stepped into the vehicle. His normal 160-pound, well-developed frame — now reduced to 129 pounds — was pathetic and gangly, nothing but skin and bones.

When we drove away from the hospital, Gary seemed really aware and happy to be going home. Sixty-five miles later, as we entered Escanaba, it was apparent that Gary recognized both the town as well as our home by the high school.

Later on, however, he displayed some strange behavior. He awakened in the morning and wondered why we changed the walls and furniture around during the night.

On Monday, the therapists questioned Gary about his weekend at home. He accused them of lying or trying to trick him. "I haven't been home in years," he retorted.

Because of Gary's reputation for antagonism, most medical staff were cautious. Breaking with the normal routine, speech therapists conducted sessions in Gary's room, apparently not wanting to risk being alone with him in their office. Some days he simply yelled, "Get the hell out of here!" and they left. He missed many therapy sessions that way.

Sometimes he was unintentionally funny. Gary's sister Vicki and her husband Dave occasionally spent the weekend with Gary to allow us a respite. One day, Dave videotaped a therapy session, listening while the speech therapist questioned Gary.

"Let's talk about your family," she said.

"How many brothers and sisters do you have?"

"One brother and one sister."

"Are they married?"

"Yes"

"Do you know what I mean when I say 'spouse'?"

"Yes, it's when you're marriage partners."

"Very good, Gary! That's excellent! Can you tell me the name of Vicki's husband?" After a long pause, Gary pleadingly looked at Dave — who is Vicki's husband — and said, "Come on, dumb-dumb! Can't you help me out here? What's her husband's name?"

The staff administered Haldol, a mind-altering drug, on what seemed to be an all-too-regular basis. In retrospect, I wonder if it was for Gary's benefit, or to provide a more pleasant working environment for themselves.

I noticed that Gary began, very frequently, to open his mouth and chew on his tongue. At first, I thought it was another residual from his injury. Later, I learned that this strange movement of the mouth and tongue was Tardive dyskinesia, a documented side effect of the Haldol. I also discovered from medical journals that Haldol is not the drug of choice for brain injured people; among other things, it can result in counterproductive reactions, leading to the very hallucinations it is prescribed to prevent.

While Gary had been making some gains with his incontinence, it began to worsen, no doubt because of the drugs he was taking.

Sometimes, the medics had to hold him down while they administered more Haldol in shot form. He would become frightened. In the face of overpowering force, Gary eventually stopped resisting.

Another new word entered my vocabulary: "perseveration." It means to fixate on one word, idea, or task, without the ability to switch back and forth or go on to the next word, idea, or task. Gary perseverated on showers. He would take as many as six to eight showers a day.

One day, neither Gary Senior nor I was able to be at the hospital, and an incident occurred. Now that Gary could get around on his own, he frequently went out to the nursing desk to ask questions. Apparently on this particular day, he wasn't satisfied with the response, or perhaps there wasn't a response. In anger, he pushed some books off the top desk onto a computer below. I received a phone call: "Gary has had a violent episode and damaged a computer."

I rushed back to the hospital. My intention was to take Gary home. They were planning to discharge him in two days anyway, about the time his insurance expired. I slept in his hospital room that night.

After a staff meeting, they recommended we give serious consideration to institutionalizing Gary. A phone conference was scheduled with Kris. They contended that "Gary could be dangerous, and a threat to children."

A very compassionate doctor visited us in Gary's room. "Take Gary home," he said. "If he has any chance of progress it will be in a home environment."

We took Gary home to Escanaba and made arrangements for him to return to his family in Kansas. Vicki, Dave, and I drove Gary to Milwaukee's airport, where Kris flew to meet us. Gary was excited when he saw Kris, kissing and hugging her before they boarded the plane to return to Kansas.

Kris said their trip was uneventful. Gary tolerated the plane ride to Wichita and then the two-hour drive to Great Bend.

The first few times I called their Kansas home, Kris reported that everything was going fairly well. Friends were helping out by taking Gary to a health club every day. They reported minimal periods of agitation.

Then, about three weeks after Gary had returned to Kansas, Kris called with a disturbing report. "Gary is in the Larned State Hospital 40 miles from here," she said. "We had an incident."

She explained further. "I try to do normal things with him. We went to a restaurant for dinner. He became loud and threw his wedding ring on the floor. We returned home, and in my frustration, I called a friend to discuss the situation. After listening to my conversation, Gary snatched the car keys and drove away. I called the police. We followed him up and down streets. Amazingly, he drove carefully, stopping at all the stop signs. The police finally encouraged him to go to the hospital emergency room. He told them he was being held hostage and had to get away. He was upset and refused to come home with me."

Since Kris could not convince Gary to return home and the local hospital was ill-equipped to handle a "psychiatric patient," the police took him to Larned State Hospital, a facility for the mentally disturbed.

"We can't leave Gary in a state mental institution — he doesn't belong there!" I said, exasperated by this turn of events. Kris was also extremely upset. We both knew the facility was inappropriate for a person with a brain injury.

After talking to Kris, I called Gary at the institution. "Please, Mom, get me out of here," he said. "Why am I here?"

Later, I obtained records from the state hospital. They included this entry:

CHIEF COMPLAINT: Patient is aggressive and hostile toward wife.

ADMISSION PSYCHIATRIC EXAMINATION: The patient appeared older than his stated age. He was dressed and groomed appropriately. He had suspicious, angry, and tense facial expressions. His behavior was withdrawn and psychomotor retardation was present. His mood was angry, with inappropriate affect. Speech was slurred and incoherent. He was disoriented to three spheres, with impaired recent and remote memory.

ASSESSMENT OF DANGEROUSNESS: He appeared to be dangerous to himself due to inability to care for himself.

COURSE AND PROGRESS OF PATIENT'S TREATMENT AND PATIENT'S RESPONSE TO TREATMENT: The patient was observed to be disoriented and confused when he was brought to the hospital on 4/20/88 at 9:00 p.m. No behavioral problems, however, were noted while he was on the ward. The patient was prescribed medication as he was before (Colace, Inderol, Tegretol, Mevacor, Haldol). The patient was discharged the following morning because the District Court had decided not to file for probable cause hearing as per arrangement with his family doctor.

ASSESSMENT OF MENTAL STATUS AT TIME OF RELEASE: Essentially, no significant change of mental status from 12 hours ago. The patient was fairly oriented to time and place. He exhibited poor comprehension and ability to express himself. His memory and insight appeared grossly impaired.

PROGNOSIS: Poor, due to nature of his illness.

TO WHOM RELEASED: To his family.

Dave volunteered to fly to Wichita to meet Gary and bring him back to Michigan. Dave was strong and would be better able to handle Gary should he become aggressive. There was another factor, too: not only were Dave and Gary brothers-in-law, they were buddies even before Dave met Gary's sister Vicki.

When Gary's tragedy occurred, it affected Dave profoundly. The two of them were like brothers. Dave, like Gary, was a 60's hippie. Sporting long black hair, a bearded face, and a placard, he once stood on Main Street in Escanaba protesting the Vietnam War. Dave also played drums in a rock band, traveling all over the Lake Michigan region to perform. Back then, Gary Senior teasingly — but affectionately — referred to him as "the wolf man." His sometimes unconventional behavior concerned and mystified his elderly parents.

Now, years later, a more conservative Dave had become a good provider and family man, with a shorter mane than Gary Senior's, and a loyalty to Gary that caused him to cross several states to retrieve his buddy from a state asylum in Kansas and bring him back to Michigan.

I remember that day well. It was my 55th birthday. Vicki baked a birthday cake while we awaited Dave and Gary's arrival. I was tense, not knowing what to expect. Had Gary's condition deteriorated? Was he dangerous? Kris and the boys would be moving back to Michigan in a month. Could we handle Gary at home?

When they arrived, Gary behaved appropriately, and kissed me on the cheek. "Happy birthday, Mom!" Again, our hopes temporarily rose.

We had some incidents the following month, however. One day my husband was late getting home from our dry cleaning business. I was getting ready to take my daily four-mile walk on a bicycle path near our home. I told Gary that his dad would be home shortly, and set out on my course before it became dark. Within ten minutes, I met my husband's vehicle and knew he would soon be home with Gary.

When I returned from my walk, my husband was furious. Apparently Gary was out in the driveway when he drove up, screaming and swearing: "Why have you done this to me?" He was disoriented and upset.

My husband, tired from the day and short on patience, shouted and chided me in front of Gary. His final comment was, "I can't deal with his behavior!" To give him some space,

I rushed Gary off to a fast food restaurant immediately, hoping everything would settle down when we returned.

It didn't. I sat at the dining room table chatting with Gary, but he was silent. Suddenly, he pushed his chair aside and lunged toward his dad, who was sitting in the living room.

Not knowing how strong Gary might be, Gary Senior shoved him into a wall in an effort to protect himself. I screamed for Gary Senior to stop. Instinctively, I took the side of my poor compromised child.

The confrontation continued. It was out of control. I screamed at Gary Senior: "Go get the police! Leave! I'll wait here." I knew that once Gary began to accelerate, an intervention was needed. I shouted again: "Hurry! Go get the police!"

Until that moment, I hadn't been afraid of Gary. But when I said "police," he grabbed my arm. His face was twisted and angry. I, too, ran out of the house. We hurried to the police station, and explained our dilemma.

Moments later, we were back at the house. I expected the worst. Instead, Gary was in his bedroom, apparently without full memory of the incident that had taken place. He appeared calm.

The police transported Gary to the hospital. We followed. Gary told the emergency room staff that they should detain his parents. "They're both crazy," he pleaded angrily. He claimed he was in bed doing nothing when the police came. He pointed to us and declared, "They're the crazy ones. Arrest them!"

This time the admitting report said:

DATE: 5/04/88

CHIEF COMPLAINT AND PRESENT ILLNESS: Mr. Abrahamson is a 37-year-old man. He experienced cardiac arrest on October 25, 1987, after jogging in Kansas. He suffered brain damage as a result. Apparently, he has moved back to Escanaba area with his parents. He had been in rehab at Marquette General earlier this year. Tonight, he apparently became quite agitated and had an argument with his father. Details are not clear as to whether he was physically assaulted, but the police were called and he was brought into the emergency room. He is awake and alert. He is fixating on things being in 1979 and says his parents are holding him involuntarily and they need to be examined. His speech is coherent, has not had any recent trauma, and because of concern about his agitation, he is being admitted.

PHYSICAL CONDITION: Slim male, speech is articulate but gets very perturbed when I ask him simple questions. He does not know the President. He keeps fixating that it is 1979.

The next day, the nursing staff reported Gary to be extremely cooperative. He was discharged later that evening.

After that episode, Gary Senior was extremely cautious around Gary. I believe Gary sensed this. People with a brain injury sometimes develop a hyper-awareness of various forms of non-verbal communication — including subtle body language cues, fleeting facial expressions, and minor changes in voice level and intonation.

Perhaps Gary's disorientation and general inability to interact made him naturally suspicious; in any case, sending the wrong signal helped to feed his already active paranoia.

Each day, we lived in fear of yet another eruption. Managing Gary came more easily to me than to my husband. I spoke softly and lovingly, and Gary responded very appropriately when the two of us were alone. He helped me shop for groceries, and we took trips to the shopping center. I was hopeful this agitated phase would pass.

On another occasion, our four-year-old grandson Zachary, Vicki's youngest boy, stayed at our home overnight. Gary became frustrated and threatened to kill himself with a knife. I read that as a ploy for attention and proceeded to give it.

My husband, already wary of Gary, thought we should take him to the psychiatric unit at Marquette General for evaluation and treatment of suicidal tendencies. When I refused, Gary Senior left the house and spent the night sleeping on the floor at our dry cleaning plant. Zachary and I stayed home with Gary. Before bedding down, we made sure to lock the bedroom door. During the night, Gary pounded on the door a couple of times before retreating to his bedroom, where he slept through the night.

I can't remember what caused the next blow up between Gary and his father, but Gary grabbed a steak knife and threatened to kill himself. After the police came, we again found ourselves in the hospital emergency room.

This time Gary stayed in the hospital for a few days, attending speech and physical therapy sessions while we waited for Kris and the boys to arrive from Kansas.

I was relieved when Kris arrived, hoping that together, as a family, we could handle Gary's behavior a little better. Anticipating her arrival, I had applied for a subsidized townhouse for Kris and Gary only blocks from our home. A June vacancy now looked possible. Gary, Kris, and the boys stayed at a small cottage on Lake Michigan, awaiting availability of their townhouse.

The townhouse was newly carpeted, sparkling clean, and, with Kris' creative flair, soon became a warm and cozy place for their family. Gary helped her arrange pictures. Kris always claimed he could arrange furniture, pictures, and flowers as well as — and sometimes better — than she.

Before his cardiac arrest, Gary had begun to focus his creative abilities on a new-found interest, photography. His Kansas job as school photographer led him to explore all types of photography, and he won awards for his Kansas landscapes. Today, three of his photos are proudly displayed in his room.

In addition to his schooling and photography, Gary also worked at a neighborhood business he had organized with Arlo, his oldest son. They mowed, raked, and cleaned up yards, working under the blazing hot Kansas sun. I sometimes wonder whether Gary experienced chest pains, or other warnings, while engaged in such physical activity.

Outside the townhouse, there was room to park the truck and camper they had used on Colorado camping trips. But the new townhouse had one problem — a prohibition against pets. Gary's pride and joy were his toy poodles, Pepper and Chantilly Lace (or Tilly for short). But the management was firm, and the dogs would have to go. The question was, go where?

Luckily, my neighbors were animal lovers; not only that, they were toy poodle lovers! They grieved over the loss of their last poodle, vowing not to get attached to another one, but they couldn't resist Tilly and Pepper. The problem of a suitable home was solved. Best of all, Gary and the boys could visit the dogs whenever they wished. It seemed as if things were going to work out for Gary and Kris.

That summer, Gary's son Leif joined a baseball league. Leif is a tremendous athlete, and baseball is one of his favorite sports. As a youngster, Gary also excelled in the sport, and more recently he played in the Great Bend church league. Gary devoted endless hours to coaching Leif, who was small for his age but very wiry and cocksure about his abilities. Leif was highly motivated, and Gary was so proud of his son's accomplishments.

Leif soon established a reputation in the league as an excellent first baseman. Though Gary may have forgotten the score, or what happened the previous inning, it did not prevent him from enjoying the *current* play.

I marveled at Gary's normalcy during those games, how he complimented Leif and gave him pointers. When we watched the game from the car, he would appropriately toot the car horn when the team scored a run.

On these and other occasions, Gary's frustration seemed nonexistent. He was relaxed, in control, and behaved appropriately to the circumstances surrounding him. It was obvious that the old Gary was, from time to time, peeking through the new one.

5

FAMILY DISCORD

Accidents will occur in the best regulated families.
- Charles Dickens

I hoped that Gary would turn a corner with the arrival of
Kris and the boys. He was back in his hometown with the
supportive strength of his entire family. Surely, progress was
inevitable.

But something was amiss. After a while, Gary seemed to
be unhappy at home. Gary's townhouse and our home were
separated by two blocks of high school property. That summer Gary wore a path crossing that field behind the high school.
He seemed to feel more comfortable at our home.

As the summer of 1988 wore on, the problem — whatever
it was — grew. He called us several times each day, and the
opening words were always the same. Speaking slowly but
urgently, he pleaded: "Please, Mother, I have got to see you.
Please. . ."

On one occasion, Gary attempted to jump from a moving
car, presumably to get to our house. Sometimes I looked out
the window and observed Gary as he sauntered across the
field with his left shoulder hanging askew. I remembered Gary
as he used to be — straight, tall, physically fit — and the tears
fell spontaneously.

One day, while we sat on the patio, he approached. On
his face was a grimace — angry and tense.

"How much do you pay that girl to stay with me?"

"Do you mean Kris?" I asked, puzzled.

"*That girl* is *not* Kris. She's an impostor!"

What was going on? He had recognized Kris up to this
point. He continued to know the boys, but for a time, Kris

was *that girl*, paid to stay with him.

During Gary's previous hospitalization phase, he had been so agitated that formal diagnostic testing — to determine the extent and nature of his brain injury — was never performed. Now seemed to be a good time to take him to Green Bay for neuropsychological testing.

At the initial intake procedure, I asked, "Why is Gary suddenly insisting that Kris is an impostor?" The neuropsychologist forwarded this theory: "Gary's wife probably isn't able to interact with him in the same way as she did before the trauma." Gary's perceptions were keen; Kris had already revealed her feelings to at least one family member: "Gary is no longer the person I married. He's a different person."

I also briefed the doctor on Gary's preoccupation with suicide threats. On many occasions Gary said, "I wish I was dead." After exhaustive testing and a lengthy discussion, the neuropsychologist reported the following:

> In summary, the patient is showing gross impairment in memory functioning consistent with his [brain injury due to oxygen deprivation]. His executive capabilities and complex problem-solving skills would also appear severely impaired. Verbal intelligence and visuospatial capabilities, as well as concentrational skills, would appear moderately impaired. Behaviorally, the patient is quite flat in his affect, but his mother has reported that he has voiced suicide ideation and is depressed .... The patient's impairments in verbal intelligence and visuospatial functioning would seem to implicate widespread, diffuse cortical involvement.
>
> I discussed these test results at much length with the patient's mother, as well as their implications. At this point, nearly nine months [since his cardiac arrest], the prognosis would appear quite guarded. Unfortunately, it is quite probable that the patient's cognitive impairments are taking on a more chronic character, though of course it is possible that he will show some improvement in the months ahead. However, it remains questionable how much possible improvement will benefit the patient functionally. The overall outlook does not appear encouraging. The patient's mother states that she is indeed seeing gains in the past

couple of months, and hopefully such gains will continue, even if they are slight. Nevertheless, a realistic appraisal of the situation would certainly appear necessary, and I tried to stress this with the patient's mother.

It is recommended that the patient continue receiving occupational therapy, speech therapy, and physical therapy in his home town. I think that we should continue these treatment programs until the patient definitely plateaus. The patient's mother will be contacting me in one month to report on any progress, and I will formally retest the patient in approximately three months. I would also strongly recommend that the patient be referred for counseling, particularly since he is voicing suicide ideation. I discussed this with the patient's mother, and she assured me that she would be contacting a counselor in the patient's home town. I also recommended to the patient's mother that she herself seek counseling, since the emotional strain on her is understandably very great. We will be discussing possible alternative living arrangements for the patient as it is indicated in the months ahead.

I drove home from Green Bay on automatic pilot. The doctor's report echoed over and over in my head. *The prognosis is guarded...cognitive impairments are taking on a more chronic character...overall outlook does not appear encouraging...a realistic appraisal is required.*

My hopes for Gary's improvement seemed to be evaporating. Tears flowed. "Why are you crying, Mom?" Gary asked, but I couldn't answer him.

As we neared home, I told Gary, "Kris is waiting for your return." *That girl*, I tried to reassure him, *really is* Kris! He wanted to believe me, it seemed, but remained skeptical.

"She'll welcome you with open arms," I said.

Unfortunately, that didn't happen. At the time, I was rankled that Kris wasn't more enthusiastic. The disappointing medical prognosis made me particularly sensitive and distressed over Gary's bleak future. I blurted, "Gary's been anxious to get home. He needs a kiss and a hug!"

That summer, I enrolled in a psychology class at our local community college. I needed to fill my mind with something other than the nightmare I was living.

Toward the middle of the summer, Gary's favorite uncle Glenn and his wife Alexis arrived in Escanaba. They spent every summer camped on the edge of Little Bay de Noc near our home. Theirs was a loving, respectful, but odd relationship because of the polarity in their ages: Glenn was 63; Alexis, 29.

Glenn met Alexis in Chicago at the home of a mutual acquaintance. Alexis was about 16. Her mother had died in childbirth, and her father had given her to a Greek family to raise. Glenn and Alexis talked often. A deep friendship developed. She confided in Glenn about some abuse she was suffering. Glenn rescued her in a frenzy, unmindful of any consequences that might result. They went to California. Glenn guided Alexis through high school. He encouraged her to continue her education. She obtained a bachelor's degree, then a master's degree, and ultimately a Ph.D. in education. Glenn beamed with pride at her accomplishments, as a father would over his daughter. I don't know when the romantic relationship blossomed, but twelve years after first meeting, they married.

Alexis is of Greek descent, with huge brown eyes and shining brown hair cropped close to her youthful, round, glowing face. She doted on every word Glenn said. Glenn, for his part, adored her.

Just before they visited, Alexis had defended her dissertation, and now she could bask in her accomplishments.

In the past they visited Gary and Kris often. Glenn was always close to our children — Gary, Vicki, and Jeff. He spent several months at a time living with us when the kids were young.

Both Glenn and Alexis loved Gary and wanted to play a part in his recovery. Gary responded well to Glenn's keen sense of humor. They treated Gary just as they had before the trauma. Gary seemed to have a sixth sense about those things, and more of Gary's old personality seemed to peep through when Glenn was around. Glenn and Alexis spent time at the apartment that Gary and Kris shared. Glenn loved being around Gary's sons.

After a while, he began to express some concern about Gary's home environment. I didn't want to believe him. I took out my rage on my husband: "Why is your brother stirring up trouble? This is the last thing we need!"

Later Alexis joined the fray, expressing concern that the calendar Gary so needed for orientation was not displayed for him to see. Gary was perseverating on his age and the year. Whenever I would see him or whenever he would call, he urgently asked, "What is my age? What year is it?" When we were in the car, he scanned license plates looking for evidence of the correct year. "How can it be 1988?" He insisted it was 1979.

One day, Kris and Gary visited Glenn and Alexis at the campground. Gary was preoccupied, wanting to visit with us instead. He told them that he wanted to leave and began walking on a road toward town. "Gary's leaving! Aren't you going to go get him?" Alexis asked. "No," Kris responded, "just let him go," as she continued to clean the glove compartment.

Clearly, the situation had become very stressful for all of us, particularly Kris. No relationship was unaffected by the strain. Soon, the thin alliance Kris and I had built during Gary's hospitalization quickly began to erode. I started to more critically observe the situation. My main concern was my son.

Sometimes, at 1:00 or 2:00 a.m., Gary would call and wake us up: "Please, Mom, I need to talk to you." I would rush over in my nightgown. One time, as we drove away from his house, he saw Kris standing in the window. "She doesn't care about me," he lamented. I tried to convince him otherwise. I took him home, put him to bed, and for a few hours, he seemed content.

One time, Kris called: "I can't manage Gary; can he spend the night with you?" When they arrived, I opened the door, Gary came in and quickly shut the door in Kris' face. I said, "Gary, say good night to Kris," trying to encourage social graces, not fully aware that, in *his* mind, she wasn't treating him right. In *his* mind, she had become *the enemy.*

On another occasion, I took Gary to the Driver's License Bureau. It took him one and a half hours to answer 50 questions. I sat near him to keep him on task. What a feat! He passed his test with flying colors and received a Michigan driver's license. The same man that doesn't know the current year or the President's name correctly answered almost all questions on a driving exam. This apparent contradiction revealed new insights into the often puzzling domain of brain injury. It showed that, despite widespread damage, a part of Gary's brain was capably functioning — and functioning well. Excited about his accomplishment, we rushed to tell Kris. She stated, "He's not driving my car. Let him drive yours."

I was finding it increasingly difficult to communicate with Kris.

Driving from their home in suburban New York, Jeff, my other son, and his wife Peggy visited that summer. Jeff was anxious to witness Gary's progress. The last time Jeff visited, Gary was still in a coma. Peggy's only face-to-face memory of Gary was at her wedding.

At the time, Peggy was a newspaper reporter. An upstate New York native, she fell in love with our area. On this trip, she wanted to go to Door County, Wisconsin. Previously we had told her all about it — the quaint shops, the delicious fish boils, artists' works on display, and sailing over miles of water.

Jeff, Peggy, Gary Senior, Gary, and I piled into our van for the three-hour trip to Door County. I sat in the back with Gary and attempted to keep him in the conversation. While the rest of them chatted incessantly, playing catch-up, I tried to occupy Gary as best I could. The trip seemed longer than three hours. Of course, I was always on pins and needles in anticipation of another eruption — possibly one we wouldn't be able to control.

We spent the day taking in the charming scenery before stopping for dinner at the White Gull Inn in Fish Creek, an historic lodge known for its unique outdoor fish boil. Peggy took pictures and astutely observed the culture. She wanted to capture aspects of the area to write about when she returned home. Peggy paints word pictures as delightful as other artists create with canvas and oils. She knows all the right colors and how to use them to her advantage.

Late that summer, my mother suffered a stroke. When she was discharged from the hospital, she came to stay with us for what was expected to be about ten days; it stretched into weeks. She and Gary were like two kids vying for my attention. When Gary visited, I probably was more attentive to him, touching off recognizable jealousy in Mom. At this point, both were egocentric.

Mom's 73rd birthday was in September. I invited about 20 family and friends over for cake. Mom, who was very ill, stayed in her bedroom.

My sister Pauline came. She managed the local country club. Gary and Kris visited her club the previous year. She was fond of "Little Gary," as she called him. Upon seeing Gary for the first time since his incident, she hugged him, then went into the back yard and cried. "He's so thin, Patt. There's no resemblance to Gary. Why us?" she lamented. "Why all these tragedies with our children?"

Pauline had suffered many tragedies in her life. She bore six children; she lost three. Paul drowned at 19 months. Debbie Jean died three days after a premature birth. And Pauline's oldest daughter Laurie succumbed to an aneurysm at age 28.

One evening, during the fall, Kris and Gary came to our house. Kris was frustrated. She confided: "Gary won't listen to me at all. Most often he is obstinate. Tonight, he wouldn't stay at a Bible class with a friend." Gary, listening to Kris' grievances, threw his Bible on the floor and left the room.

Gary Senior, the only one home at the time, sympathized with Kris. "I know it's difficult for you. It's difficult for all of us. Patt is so good at solutions. Maybe she has some ideas about where we go from here. Come and talk to her tomorrow."

I reflected on their 15-year marriage and gave some deep thought as to how I might handle this situation. A few days later, Kris and Gary came for a return visit. "Kris, I can only tell you what I would do if it were my husband needing help. Gary needs speech and occupational therapy badly. It's almost a year since his trauma." Both of us were aware of the potential benefits to early intervention. I continued, "If it were me, I'd sell Gary's camper and truck. They're just sitting there idle. It would give you the co-payment you need so Gary can receive Medicaid. He could get the therapy he needs so badly. Maybe now he would be more receptive to various forms of therapy."

We were in the kitchen. After a short, terse exchange of words, Kris declared, "I'm not selling everything I own!" and headed for the door. "This is *your* husband we're talking about," I said. Visibly shaken and probably nervous about her future and that of her boys, she offered a final, parting statement: "Why don't you sell your house if you want to help?!"

Poor Gary sat bewildered in the kitchen. He ran to the door. Nervously, he yelled, "Hey! Hey! Stop that!" This marked the end of any cohesion between Kris and me.

Gary Senior would have one more volatile exchange of words with her: "Gary is *your* husband. He is legally and morally *your* responsibility." Unfortunately, the stress and uncertainty were creating rifts when we most needed togetherness.

In November, my mother died. Kris attended the funeral with Gary. Kris and I spoke to one another only when absolutely necessary.

Gary Senior and I continued to pick up Gary daily. Arlo, Gary's oldest son, became the go-between for us. When further communication between Kris and I was necessary, Gary — playing the role of carrier pigeon — unknowingly carried notes in his pocket. The situation had become bizarre. In all this, Gary was the loser.

Arlo seemed deeply affected by the change in his father, of his misaligned form that was once so perfect, of his unusual behavior in public. All his life he had looked up to this man, felt proud of him.

Unfortunately, some of Arlo's high school peers helped fuel any embarrassment he may have been feeling. When they saw Gary crossing the field, they'd say (seemingly with malice): "There goes that retard again."

For a while, Gary Senior attended Arlo's basketball games. The breakdown in communication was evident, as Gary Senior sat in one area, and Gary and Kris sat in another. Sometimes, Gary would leave Kris and join his father if he spotted him in the bleachers. Finally, Gary Senior decided to stop going to the games he enjoyed so much, because of the deepening rift in our relationship with Kris.

One day, in the spring of 1989, we were unable to reach Gary. Since I spent time with him every day, I was very concerned. Four days later, Arlo explained that they had been visiting relatives in Chicago. I found out later that they had taken Gary to Grand Rapids for an evaluation that might lead to a scholarship providing in-patient treatment.

We were encouraged by this undertaking. We had begun to worry what would happen to Gary. Since he apparently was no longer deemed to be a functioning family member, we thought his days at home might be numbered.

Ultimately, Gary did not get the scholarship. It had been well over one year since Gary's traumatic brain injury. The selection committee apparently decided that others with less acute, and more recent, brain injuries would make better candidates.

Outside, freezing rain pounded on the windows. The doorbell rang. It was 8:00 or 9:00 p.m. Who could it be? Horrified, I saw Gary standing alone outside the lead glass door of the foyer. He was scantily dressed, soaking wet, and icy cold to touch. His hands were purple and his face was red. Urine was running down his legs. My poor boy was shaking uncontrollably. He remembered that he had walked across the main highway from Kris' brother's house, a distance of almost three miles.

As the story unfolded, Arlo appeared at our door about one hour later. He explained, "We were visiting my uncle and Dad wanted to leave. He went to sit in the car, like he often does. I went out to check on him. He was gone."

Gary spent that night with us.

Glenn had been urging me to call the Adult Protective Services Division of the Michigan Department of Social Services. Now, I too had a heightened concern for Gary's welfare.

I was aware that Kris — and I assumed Gary too — were receiving services at the Community Mental Health Center. Perhaps I could voice my concerns to these professionals. But when I tried, I was discreetly informed, "I cannot discuss this case with you. It would breach our confidentiality policy."

"But it's my son," I pleaded.

The psychologist remained unfazed, so I told her, "You leave me no other alternative than to call Adult Protective Services."

The frequency of phone calls from Gary escalated. He'd call at midnight, 1:00 a.m., 2:00 a.m. — all hours of the night.

One night, my husband insisted that we disconnect the phone to get some much-needed rest. The following day, a Sunday, we picked Gary up in the afternoon to have dinner with us. Something was different. He was lethargic, almost as if he'd been drugged. He slept several hours at our house during the afternoon, before dinner.

That evening, a church member called: "Are you aware that your son was taken to the hospital last night? I don't know the details; something about a knife and suicide. Kris' sister was talking about it in church this morning."

My mind reeled. No wonder he was so lethargic. He *had* been drugged — at the hospital! I felt profoundly sad. Gary had no doubt tried to call us in his desperation. I felt so upset that I wasn't there for him when he needed me.

This newly discovered information was unsettling. But before I could act on it, I received a call from the local Community Mental Health office: "I am scheduling a meeting for all persons interested in Gary's welfare and future. Come to this office on Wednesday at 5:00 p.m."

Wednesday came. The date was May 7, 1989, eighteen months after Gary's trauma, but it seemed like a lifetime. Early in the day, I had my last final exam at school. I had to temporarily brush aside the overriding concern in my life — Gary — and study to get through my exam.

Just before 5:00 p.m., Vicki, Dave, Gary Senior, and I waited in the lobby for the meeting to convene, a meeting that was sure to culminate in drastic changes for all of us.

The psychologist asked us to follow her into a crowded lounge-type room. Gary, Kris, Kris' brother, and Kris' sister sat mute, appearing tense, at the far end of the room. When we came in, Gary got up and moved to sit by Dave.

I remember thinking: *Why are Kris' brother and sister*

here? I thought this meeting was for Gary's advocates. Certainly, they aren't in his camp. Months earlier, Kris had seemed irritated with her family's dissenting comments — encouraging her to let go, to leave Gary.

Gary sat quietly as the crisis intervention meeting began. The psychologist got right to the point. "The reason for this meeting is to discuss Gary's future." Although we already knew of his recent suicide threat, the psychologist provided additional details: "This past weekend, Gary took a butcher knife out of the drawer and announced he was going to kill himself. Police were called, and Gary was rushed to the hospital .... Kris cannot restrain Gary .... He perseverates, wanting to be at his parents' home regardless of the hour ..."

Sitting motionless, my eyes fixed on the speaker, I silently began to editorialize: *Suicide threats are a desperate, serious call for help. Perhaps Gary's desire to be at our home is not merely perseverative; maybe it's not motivated by some sort of pathological compulsion toward nonproductive repetition. It could be meaningful behavior. Perhaps he sees our home as a haven where he's treated more like the old Gary.*

The psychologist continued: "Gary is no longer able to reside at home with his wife and sons .... The need for treatment has been explored. Because Gary does not have the funds to purchase private rehabilitative care, his options include involuntary hospitalization or a convalescent facility."

Kris' brother spoke up: "Nobody — nobody in this room including myself could handle this situation for one week, let alone one year."

Gary became extremely nervous. An institution or a convalescent home? He heard. He understood. He stood up and attempted to leave. Dave accompanied him into the hallway. Gary may have had trouble communicating in words, but he could take action. All his instincts told him to get away.

I felt relieved once Gary left the room. Poor Gary — a husband, a father, a son, a brother; now he had been reduced to *a problem.* Why were we discussing his behavior and his prospects right in front of him — as if he were a nonperson, someone without personal feelings or fears? Was there no compassion?

The psychologist recommended, as an immediate step,

that we take Gary home for the weekend to give Kris some respite until additional decisions could be made.

At that point, I already knew that we had to exercise the obvious third choice: Gary Senior and I would care for him until a better option could be determined. Institutionalization must be the last resort. I knew that Gary would simply degenerate in the institutions under consideration. We would search out and consider other alternatives.

Gary, Gary Senior, Vicki, Dave, and I proceeded down the hall to leave the premises. Kris attempted a weak overture toward Gary. He seemed to purposefully ignore her and step up his pace to get away as we left the building.

For all practical purposes, Gary and Kris' marriage, sadly, had ended.

6

GARY MOVES HOME

Home is the place where,
when you have to go there,
they have to take you in.
              - Robert Frost

We drove away from the Mental Health Center meeting in silence, each consumed with private thoughts.

I was angry with myself. During the meeting, we addressed the question of whether Gary Senior and I would be willing, through a legal guardianship, to be Gary's permanent caretakers. We agreed to consider it. We were noncommittal. Gary, who had suffered so, would have been there for us in time of need. Now his closest family members could only *think about* whether or not they wanted to oversee his future.

I was angry with my husband. In our conversation before the meeting, we anticipated events would turn out exactly as they did. When I posed the question of "What if . . .," my husband adamantly opposed Gary's coming to live with us permanently.

Lastly, I was angry with Kris. At the time, I wondered how she could abandon her husband like this. In retrospect, we probably expected too much from Kris. Dana Reeve, the wife of movie actor Christopher Reeve, suggested that her decision to stick by her husband after his horse riding accident — which left him paralyzed — was made easier because he was still the person she knew and loved, there was "no head injury, no brain damage." Despite his physical condition, she said, he was still "him, the essence of him."

With severe brain injury, however, "until death do us part" may not always be realistic. Kris loved the old Gary; the new

Gary was a stranger to her, and she a stranger to him. More-over, Kris had the welfare of her boys to think about. It may have been different, for example, had Gary developed a brain abnormality from Alzheimer's in retirement years, long after the children were fully grown. Instead, Kris was all at once confronted with Gary's bizarre behavior, the duties of parent-hood, and the responsibility of managing a household on a limited income. It was probably too much for Kris to handle.

When you lose a loved one through death, the family goes through a grieving process but then moves on. By contrast, when you lose a loved one through brain injury, the family goes through a similar grieving process but is also faced with issues of 24-hour care, bizarre behavior, and financial pres-sures, all of which can trigger intra-family squabbles. These squabbles, in turn, tend to increase everyone's stress. It's a vicious cycle.

In the end, Kris felt constrained to focus on herself and her boys. She felt that the children were not just missing one parent (Gary) but were actually missing both parents as so much of her time, by necessity, was devoted to Gary's care.

Likewise, I focused on *my* son, whom I loved and raised. Even Gary Senior — always cautious and on guard, not quite trusting the new Gary — was there for him, a good father to his son. The bond between a parent and child is so special that, once formed, nothing can break it. While a spouse can walk away, a parent cannot. Gary *was* coming home, even if only temporarily, until I could find a more suitable placement.

On the way home, Vicki broke the silence: "Why don't we go to Pizza Hut? None of us has had dinner yet."

While we waited for the pizza, Gary was normal, talkative and perceptibly happy.

"Mom, Gary can come and spend the weekend with us," Vicki suggested, "to give you and Dad a break."

"That's a good idea," I replied. "Gary loves to be around you and Dave."

At that time, Vicki and Dave lived 50 miles from our home. But, early in the morning after his first night at their house, Vicki called: "All Gary says is, 'I want to see my mother and dad.'" She had been up all night with him, and that's all he talked about. Within an hour of our phone conversation, we met and took Gary back home again.

Arlo brought some of Gary's clothes over. A few days went by. Now, the tables turned. Kris and the boys picked up Gary on occasion, bringing him back within an hour or two. Gary was always excited about going with them.

Because of Gary's perseveration, he was difficult to be around. He would ask his age and the year 200 to 300 times a day. The behavior seemed to accelerate when we watched TV. He was egocentric and demanded our full attention. His father's tolerance for this behavior was lower than mine. After a certain period of time, he would shout: "Gary, go to your room. You're not going to dominate us like that." In response, Gary would shake and hobble quickly out of the room yelling "I can't take this anymore." At times, Gary would continue to perseverate, to the point of needing medication to calm down. I felt caught between them again. I'd attempt to use diplomacy to calm Gary and try to reason with my husband: "Your outbursts exacerbate the situation. You have to control yourself." Many arguments ensued, then silence would prevail for days.

When we weren't arguing, I would spend time searching out help for Gary. At first, my advocacy efforts seemed futile. I'd place a call to this or that agency and be told time after time, "Someone will get back to you on this," but they never did. I'd get referred to another party in another department or at another agency, and end up chasing my tail.

I called our congressman, Bob Davis. In the past he had arranged an internship for our son Jeff as a legislative aide. In turn, I had acted as his campaign co-chair for several years. He knew our family personally; surely he would help us.

He intervened by placing a personal call to the Director of the Michigan Department of Social Services. Almost immediately, I received a call from the Director's office: "We will contact Mary Free Bed Hospital in Grand Rapids. The hospital has a traumatic brain injury unit. He will need to have an evaluation there. If he qualifies, he would be included in a pilot program of 15 individuals, all residents of Michigan, who are victims of traumatic brain injury. The transitional living program would be geared toward eventual employment and independent living."

I couldn't believe my ears. Finally, someone was going to help us! "When can I expect to bring Gary to Grand Rapids?" I asked.

"The hospital will contact you and make all the arrangements. The evaluation will take about three weeks."

I hung up. Our prayers for help had been answered. I quickly called my husband to inform him of the great news.

Glenn and Alexis came for the summer, as usual. Alexis had secured a teaching position at Eureka College, a private university in Illinois and President Reagan's alma mater. She was pleased with her first paying job.

Both Glenn and Alexis were very supportive and seemed pleased that Gary was with us. They sent Gary frequent letters and cards. They came to spend time with him and to help out. They had observed a great difference in Gary compared to the summer before. His weight near normal now, Gary's face was no longer sunken and etched with lines. They also commented, on the negative side, how the perseveration had increased from the summer before. Gary perseverated incessantly on his age, everyone else's age, and the year. He constantly repeated: "I've lost my job and everything."

Glenn lived in Grand Rapids at one time, so he was aware of Mary Free Bed Hospital. He gave us some encouragement about what we might expect there.

While we waited for the call from Mary Free Bed, we arranged to have Gary placed in a physical therapy program, funded through Michigan Rehabilitation Services, at a local hospital. I would drop him off at the hospital and, in an effort to promote independence, have him take a cab home (with assistance from hospital staff).

On the days he had physical therapy, I noticed he returned home agitated, often remaining in that mood for the rest of the day. Later, I discovered that one male therapist was confrontational and used force to direct Gary's actions. Up until that time, the staff had only limited experience with brain injury survivors. Gary lacked motivation due to the brain injury; he also lacked energy as a result of his untreated heart condition. They apparently attributed these behavioral characteristics to mere laziness. With a little experimentation, they'd have found progress was possible with a gather-more-bees-with-honey-than-vinegar approach. Seeing very little progress and witnessing Gary's increased agitation after these sessions, I discontinued the therapy, hoping to find more appropriate direction from the staff in Grand Rapids.

Before the tragedy, Gary liked to jog and be physically active. In place of the physical therapy sessions, I initiated a walking program on the bicycle path near our home. He seemed to tire easily, though. After walking four or five blocks, he would become short of breath and want to go home. Once at home, he often retreated to his bed.

Not yet realizing the full ramifications of Gary's memory problem, I worked to foster independence in him — to prepare him for re-entry into the community. We live only four blocks from a shopping plaza. Sometimes I dropped Gary off, told him that there was a note in his pocket with our phone number and instructions to call when he wanted to return home. Due to short-term memory problems, Gary never remembered to look in his pocket. However, due to his less impaired long-term memory, he *did* remember where we lived and could walk home. Once at the shopping plaza, he'd enter the bookstore — where our dry cleaning business was once located — and ask where his mother and father were. Just minutes after I dropped him off, he'd look the store attendant in the eye and declare: "I haven't seen my mom and dad in five years."

I also tried sending him to the doughnut shop three blocks away to buy his favorite chocolate-frosted treat. It was a bit risky to expect that he'd remember to cross the busy intersection only on a green light. But, then again, the skills needed to safely cross a street didn't really implicate short-term memory, one of his primary deficits. Moreover, if I didn't allow him some latitude, he perceived himself as "locked up," as if we were holding him prisoner.

I'll always remember the day he returned from the doughnut shop, clutching a white doughnut shop bag as he headed up our driveway. It had taken him four tries, but he had done it! His dad and I jumped up and down, kissed him, congratulated him and rejoiced in his achievement. Casting a genuinely puzzled look at us, he asked, "What's the big deal about buying a doughnut?" Clearly, he thought we were nuts!

When it came to dealing with Gary's brain injury and its ramifications, I was no more experienced than the hospital staff — a novice, learning something new about brain injury every day. I learned that Gary had a coded way of speaking, which can't be taken literally.

Whenever Gary Senior was gone for a few hours, Gary asked about him, saying he hadn't seen his dad in five years. At times, his speech was crude and crass. He would say, "I haven't taken a shit for five years." It took me a while to learn that, in fact, he was announcing his need to have a bowel movement. He complained that he hadn't eaten in ten years. That meant he was hungry.

He would ask, "How are you, Mom?" Then, before I could answer, he'd add "I'm lost; I've lost my job and everything." He was fixated on being "lost." If we met someone at the grocery store or shopping mall, his answer to "How are you?" was always "I'm lost." Even today, his reply is always the same. People who don't understand this are quick to respond, "Gary, you're not lost; this is Escanaba."

One day, I tried to elicit from him what he meant by the word "lost." He replied, "Lost in time — I don't know what my age is, what year it is, or anything." I thought, *What a profound statement.* From that moment on, I realized that Gary *really was* lost: lost in time and space.

We drove by gas stations with the price per gallon marked prominently and Gary would exclaim in amazement how high the price of gas was. Or when we went to the drive-through window of a fast food restaurant, he would repeat the price in disbelief, claiming highway robbery. He compared everything to 1979, the year he fixed on when he emerged from the coma. Yes, Gary truly was lost in time and space.

It took time before I understood why Gary didn't care to watch TV for longer than a minute or two. He couldn't follow a story because he couldn't remember what happened five minutes before. Occasionally, if there was a steamy sex scene, his attention span was a bit longer. He didn't enjoy reading for the same reason: he couldn't remember the previous page.

Gary *did* remember old TV shows like *Bonanza, Dennis the Menace, Father Knows Best,* and *I Love Lucy.* He also knew every rock band that was popular during the 1960's and 1970's, along with song lyrics from those years, especially Beatles' songs. Sometimes he cried when he heard certain songs; perhaps the music was a cue, triggering special memories. Sensitive to his pain, feeling helpless to fix it, I cried at those times, too.

His memory of songs, bands, and TV shows was heartening; yet he remembered little of his high school graduation. And, there was no memory of his graduation from the community college in Kansas. Oxygen deprivation had apparently wiped out the memory trace.

We found, as a rule, most of his memories from 1980 to the trauma date in 1987 are virtually erased from his mind. Memories from 1978 and before remain largely in tact, with some exceptions. And memories from 1979 — a year that apparently marks some mysterious dividing line in his brain — are episodal, sporadic, and sketchy. His son Leif was born that year; sometimes he remembers, sometimes not.

On good days, Gary *did* have *some* short-term memory function. He was able to encode and store certain short-term memories, but unable to properly categorize them for accurate retrieval. For example, I would say, "You have an appointment with Dr. So-and-So tomorrow." Later, I asked, "What was that doctor's name?" He would mention two or three — all valid names of doctors he'd seen recently — but not necessarily the right one.

Gary had both retrograde amnesia (unable to recall certain events before the trauma) as well as post-traumatic amnesia (difficulty learning new skills and remembering events after the trauma).

In addition to memory trouble, the cardiac arrest left Gary with a number of other problems, including limited physical strength and agility, perseveration, and low motivation. But, it seemed the memory problem would be one of his biggest hurdles to independence.

The neuropsychologist determined that Gary has severe damage to the hippocampus area of the brain, an integral part of his memory system. This translates to living in permanent limbo. Little is known about whether other areas of the brain can take over for this damaged area. There are no simple formulas to treat memory problems.

Nevertheless, I learned all I could about memory, determined to ferret out every possible detail that would help me understand what was happening to my son. Ironically, it seemed the more I read and learned, the less I *really* understood; it was all so puzzling and complex.

I did learn this: memory holds together our experiences. It gives us proper context to guide future actions. I tried to place myself in Gary's position, to conceive of *not* remembering what happened last year, last week, yesterday, or even fifteen minutes before. Without short-term memory, life would be confusing, frightening, even utterly meaningless; every experience would be a first then dissipate, like a sudden flash of a firework burst, bright for the moment, but then fading before completely disappearing. It would be puzzling because you could not reflect on the past, you could not learn from it, you could not make plans for the future. Life would be episodal, discrete, little sets of moments, soon forgotten. Gary's description of himself as "lost in time and space" seems eerily precise. No wonder he got agitated. Memory loss left him disoriented, making the world around him seem surreal, like a jumbled confusion.

Armed with growing knowledge, I began to question the accuracy of the specialists' still-negative prognosis. Gary had no one but us to ensure he got the best possible treatment. I was convinced that my tenacity would eventually effect change in Gary.

I became engrossed in the subject of memory, looking for clues in Gary to unlock new knowledge for me. Gary loved to ride in the car. He was most relaxed while riding, scanning the scene for license plates or other evidence that it actually was the year I said it was.

When we drove by my mother's house, he would say, "How's Grandma?" I'd reply, "Grandma died last year, Gary."

He'd express shock and grief: "Oh, no! My grandma died?!" But I discovered little tricks that told me he *did* encode the information he was given, even though he was unable to retrieve it on his own. It was there, imprinted in his head somewhere. I discovered that if I asked him "Where is Grandma?" just before we drove past her house, at first he would answer "I don't know" as if he were questioning himself. Then he'd pause and say, "She died?" He *did* know, but he was unsure if his memory was accurate. It was as if the memory were at the level of intuition; he was not really sure of it. He was guessing; he thought she might be dead, but wasn't sure why he thought that.

I learned that I had to be careful with my questions. If I were too confrontational, he became agitated, shouting "I don't know!" If, on the other hand, I cued him by asking "Does this seem familiar?" he would be more willing to discuss the subject at hand. In short, Gary needed to be treated with kid gloves, something his therapists didn't always do. Direct questions intimidated him; he closed himself off to further questioning. I think his self-esteem was threatened when he found himself unable to answer a direct question. It made him feel uncomfortable and inept. Most of the time, he was in denial about his cognitive deficits; but direct questions exposed him, making him feel intellectually naked, unable to hide his deficits. Since I too was in denial about Gary's prognosis and chances for full recovery, I could relate to all this. Denial is a modulator, a protection from experiencing overwhelming trauma; denial helps us digest grossly negative information gradually, in small bits, not all at once.

I tried to explain to Gary what had happened to him. I reasoned that showing him a videotape taken while he was at Marquette General Hospital might help him recall. When he saw himself engaged in rudimentary therapies, with his face so painfully thin and his shoulders slumped, he became angry. He vehemently denied this was him. He insisted it was an impostor. The image was too painful to Gary. The man in the video simply did not match his self-image.

When he looked in a mirror, he would exclaim, "I'm old now! How old am I?" When he looked at his dad or me, he would say "You're an old man now" or "You're an old lady now, right?"   Apparently, he was comparing our current appearance to the image he had of us, his parents, in 1979.

I discovered that for Gary to eat a full meal, every bite would have to be encouraged. No wonder he was predisposed to thinness. At times, I actually had to spoon feed him. He also had a tendency to choke. A delayed swallow was evident. He held liquid in his mouth and his eyes would enlarge until it occurred to him to swallow. It was no longer automatic.

Another reason Gary cared little about meals was his diminished sense of smell, which affected his ability to taste. Sweets were all he ate readily. It took over two years before Gary could smell again. I discovered it by accident one day. I was applying a pungent after-shave lotion when he winced and said, "What's the name of that awful stuff?" Of course, I delighted in his returning sense of smell. Just like the incident with the doughnuts, he was puzzled: "What's the big deal? Can't everybody smell?"

7

MARY FREE BED

Life consists of what a man is thinking of all day.
- Ralph Waldo Emerson

In July 1989, we received a call from Mary Free Bed Hospital. Two months had passed since I was informed that Gary would be given an opportunity to qualify for one of 15 spots in a transitional living program for victims of traumatic brain injury (TBI). To determine whether Gary was an appropriate candidate for the program, he had to undergo three weeks of evaluation at Mary Free Bed Hospital.

With new hopes and expectations, we packed Gary's suitcase and left for Grand Rapids, a six-hour drive — first east, then south across the Mackinac Bridge into lower Michigan. Our game plan included spending the first few days with Gary to meet his therapists; then, we would go to Washington, D.C. and visit Jeff and Peggy for a much-needed respite. We would also visit Congressman Davis' Washington office before returning to the hospital within a week.

We entered the city of Grand Rapids and, with anticipation, made a beeline to the hospital. Once inside, my first visual impressions of Mary Free Bed's TBI unit filled me with sadness: paralyzed boys, those with empty looks, those in wheelchairs, those with futures that should have been bright. I didn't see one female victim. But, that made sense; boys are generally more physically active, more reckless, more prone to accidents that result in brain injuries. Wandering around were bewildered-looking families, searching for answers, hoping to be told, "Your boy will be all right. It just takes time."

I know now that no doctor on earth can predict the outcome of a brain injury like Gary's. We were entering a waiting game that could take years, decades, and in the end — after everything was done that could be done — genuine resolution might elude us altogether.

Still, I was impressed with the TBI unit at Mary Free Bed. The unit was in a special section of the hospital, separate from other areas.

I was also pleased with Gary's initial reaction: he wanted to cooperate, he wanted to be able to work again. "I'll do what I have to," he assured us.

His response was especially appropriate when he met his roommate, a car crash victim with a brain injury. Robert was a tall, slim, young man with glasses. Recently discharged from the military, Robert was a bit of a perfectionist. Apparently thinking he was still on base, he nervously smoothed his bedspread and showed us how to bounce a quarter on it. He told Gary, "The accommodations here are not bad, but the pay is lousy: only $30 per week." Gary gazed toward us and drew a frown. Then, cackling like the old Gary, he said, "Dad, this guy must be nuts — whoever heard of a hospital paying you to be here?"

We unpacked his clothes, got him settled, and left for a nearby motel.

At dawn the next morning, we hurried to the hospital to see how Gary fared his first night, arriving before the night shift left. The nurse said Gary did very well until he was awakened by his roommate in the middle of the night. Robert was very urgent: "Get out of bed. We're in the wrong bed. We have to change beds immediately!" Poor Gary. Perplexed in his own right, his confusion doubled as he dealt with a confused roommate.

I met with Gary's doctor that morning and expressed concern about Gary's undiagnosed heart problem. We agreed that a work-up was necessary to evaluate Gary's cardiac status. After all, a cardiac arrest is what got him into trouble in the first place.

Since Gary needed constant orientation, I made an audio tape explaining where he was, why he was there, and when we would be back from Washington, D.C. I instructed the staff to remind Gary to play the tape. I also made a sign with answers to often-asked questions and fastened it to the wall at the foot of his bed. The staff placed an ankle monitor on him for his own safety. We hugged him, bade him good-bye, and left for the nation's capital.

I might just as well have stayed with Gary, because he never left my thoughts. My husband couldn't understand my obsession. "This is what we waited for," he said. "Gary is in good hands. We're able to spend a few days away from the war zone," he reasoned. "Why can't you enjoy it?" I don't think I answered him; I just stared at the scenery rushing by as we headed east down the Ohio turnpike toward Washington, D.C.

Back at the hospital, the staff began to evaluate Gary's condition. Later, I obtained the hospital records. One report said the following:

> Gary arrived for the appointment on foot. When asked for biographical information, he gave his age and birth date, along with the city in which he was living. He indicated that he was a high school graduate with about two years of college. He did not know what year it was. He was unsure whether or not he was married anymore or with whom he was living previous to admission to Mary Free Bed. He thought he had children. When asked about his cardiac arrest, he stated that he could not remember having a heart attack. He was not sure he even had a heart attack. At this point, he became quite suspicious, implying that the examiner might have invented his diagnosis. He was oriented to person, but was clearly disoriented to time and circumstance.
>
> When asked about any symptoms he might be having following his accident, Gary denied having headaches. He also denied having any cognitive difficulties, with the exception of "a little" trouble with his memory. He denied depression. He stated that he was able to sleep at night. When asked about his appetite, he stated, "I don't know, I eat all the food." When asked about his future, he stated, "I would like to see my parents again. I haven't seen them since 1979."

Gary is a Caucasian man with brown hair who came to the appointment wearing casual pants and T-shirt. He had a rather blank facial expression and seemed somewhat disoriented. He walked with a droop to the right shoulder and a wide-based gait. Gary's spontaneous speech was slow, with short sentences. Response time to questions was fairly long, and mental processing seemed slow. He perseverated on his own age and the examiner's age periodically throughout the interview. Short-term memory was clearly impaired (e.g., in his inability to remember that he had been living with his parents). He did not initiate any topics or interactions. Thought processes appeared to be very concrete (e.g., in his description of his appetite). Affect seemed bland, except when frustrated, when he became hostile. He appeared very sensitive to possible slights. For example, when asked to recite the alphabet, he asked, in an angry fashion, "Do you think I'm stupid?"

He began masturbating in a mechanical way about halfway through the interview. When asked to stop touching himself, he became hostile and confrontational, asking the examiner what she meant. It is possible that he was not fully aware of his behavior and, in fact, he continued the behavior except when the examiner made eye contact with him.

Another report stated:

Gary has been separated from his wife, Kris, since May of 1989 at which time he went to live with his parents, Gary Senior and Patricia. His parents report that prior to the injury the marriage was stable. Gary's parents describe Gary as being generally cooperative, congenial, and pleasant. Gary's parents also report, however, that if overstimulated, Gary on occasion displays a temper. Gary's parents report that Gary has a history of being rebellious towards authority.

Gary's parents are very supportive. Patricia Abrahamson is a strong advocate for her son. Patricia has been involved with the Michigan Head Injury Alliance and is knowledgeable regarding head injury.

Upon admission Gary was confused and disoriented as to where he was, why he was here, and who the staff was around him. The plan of social work was to utilize orientation techniques and encourage family and staff to utilize notes, journals, etc. Although these strategies were utilized, Gary was not able to take significant advantage of them due to his poor short-term memory. Gary's memory was significantly impaired, and he could not become oriented to the point where it was a significant benefit to him.

Upon admission it was recognized that the patient may be having a difficult time adjusting from his recent separation from his wife and from his children. The goal of social work was to assess the patient's ability to discuss this. Social work assessed that the patient was not able to partake in significant counsel regarding these issues and that it would not be appropriate for the patient to participate in counseling at this time.

Also, upon admission, the family displayed a frustration over the lack of resources available to them to help their son. These would include Medicaid funding to support further rehabilitation of Gary. The plan by social work was to advocate for the patient and his family to the State of Michigan and to facilitate adequate funding for clinically indicated programs that the team may feel were appropriate for referral. Social work will keep in close contact with the State of Michigan regarding Medicaid funding and Gary's appropriateness to access this funding.

The report concluded that Gary would be discharged into the care of his parents should he be deemed inappropriate for the transitional living program. Since Gary Senior and I had not come up with a viable alternative, we hoped and expected that Gary would be accepted into the program.

Once in Washington, we visited Congressman Davis' office. Mark Ruge, Davis' Chief of Staff, greeted us. We knew Mark personally as a high school friend of Jeff's. We informed Mark that Congressman Davis' previous personal contact with the Michigan Department of Social Services on behalf of Gary was bearing fruit. He seemed pleased that Gary was being evaluated at Mary Free Bed Hospital for possible placement in a brain injury program. He assured us that he would pass along the good news to Congressman Davis. We thanked Mark for his efforts, exited the Rayburn House Office Building, and walked across the East Front of the Capitol Building toward the Supreme Court.

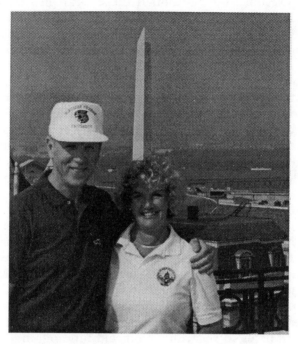

Gary Senior and Patt in Washington, DC, 1989.

Jeff had made arrangements for us to visit the Supreme Court Justices' Chambers. A staffer and friend of Peggy's from Sandra Day O'Connor's office gave us a personal tour behind the scenes. It was extremely interesting. I sat in Sandra Day O'Connor's elegant high-back chair, which dated back to the previous century. Down by my feet and at the foot of every chair was a polished brass spittoon: a throwback to the days when many gentlemen chewed tobacco. I viewed the wide expanse of the chambers and reflected on the distinguished individuals that had sat on the Court — John Marshall, Oliver Wendell Holmes, Louis Brandeis. In their wildest imagination they probably never thought a female justice would one day grace the chambers.

My thoughts were interrupted by a group tour walking through the back of the room. Suddenly, they began snapping pictures of me sitting in the chair. From a distance, they must have thought *I* was Sandra Day O'Connor, the only woman on the Supreme Court at the time. It was an awesome experience, imagining the history made in that room.

Later that day we visited the FBI Building. I remember being bored while waiting in line to enter the building, but my boredom vanished as we looked through glass cases of the unbelievable arsenal confiscated over the years. On display were guns owned by notorious criminals such as Baby Face Nelson, John Dillinger, and Lee Harvey Oswald. It was fascinating, yet I couldn't seem to really enjoy anything. My mind was constantly on Gary. I phoned the hospital several times daily, pestering the nurses and irritating my husband.

After several days in Washington, we headed back to Grand Rapids. Worried about his father's nervousness and reluctance to drive such distances, Jeff drove us back and visited his brother at the same time. We arrived in Grand Rapids late at night but postponed visiting Gary at the hospital until the morning.

Two more weeks of evaluation had yet to be completed, but what I heard from the therapists was not encouraging. Apparently, Gary was uncooperative and sometimes agitated during his first week at Mary Free Bed. To make him easier to handle, the staff placed him on drugs, which also made him lethargic. He ate little and threatened to starve himself to death.

Gary seemed pleased to see us. We took him to lunch at St. Mary's Cafeteria. In our presence, he ate adequately, if not well. Upon returning to his unit, we walked into the common area, which had a piano in the middle of the room. Jeff sat down and began to play. As a teenager, Jeff played guitar in a rock band (named "Clinton"), and on a couple of occasions Gary helped drive his band to out-of-town jobs. Suddenly, without warning, Gary exploded in a fit of frustration: "This is bullshit!" he said, getting up out of his chair. He then marched to his room and got into bed. Within five or ten minutes he calmed down, but the incident left me with an uneasy feeling.

A couple of days later, with some apprehension, we left to go back to Escanaba. Gary remained at Mary Free Bed for two more weeks of evaluation. As we drove away, I was consumed with guilt and sadness. I knew he wouldn't eat well;

and with impaired short-term memory, he probably wouldn't realize that we were coming back or even understand why he was there.

Later, I received a copy of the nursing notes, which validated most of my fears. These excerpts paint a depressing picture of Gary's unenviable, forlorn condition as well as his intense resistance to institutional living.

8/3/89

1:00 p.m. - Patient ate lunch with parents at St. Mary's Cafeteria. They report he ate well. Parents left to go home. Patient expressed fear that his parents would leave him and never come back.

6:00 p.m. - Patient found wandering on the stairs "looking for door." Was escorted back to nursing unit. Ankle monitor is on. Patient offered a shake to drink. Stated "I'm not hungry!" Patient threw the milk shake on the floor.

8/4/89

7:30 a.m. - Set up for breakfast in patient's room. Needs encouragement to eat. Insists that he is not hungry.

8/5/89

1:30 p.m. - Patient refused most of meal. Became belligerent when encouraged to eat. Wandering in hall, stated "going to find my parents." Continues agitated.

8/6/89

2:00 p.m. - Patient refused most of lunch. Patient's mother called and talked with patient.

8:00 p.m. - Mom called. Patient happy to talk to her.

8/7/89

4:00 p.m. - Patient in room stating "you'd be in a terrible mood too, if you were stuck here."

6:30 p.m. - Came out of room with coat on, walking very fast. Attempting to get "out." Went out emergency exit and escorted back in. Very angry about being here and yelling "I'll get back to Escanaba if I have to walk there and kick your ass."

7:00 p.m. - Doctor here and redirected patient by talking about Kansas and Escanaba. Received orders for agitation. Patient directed back to room and was calm for five minutes. Back out of room, attempting to leave. Swinging arms at caregivers. Threw Pepsi on floor. Swinging arms and yelling, "I'll get out of here — you just wait!" Attempted talking to mother on phone, but slammed phone down within one minute. Agitation increased. Haldol 5 mg. given for severe agitation.

7:45 p.m. - One-on-one maintained until patient calm. Family notified regarding patient's agitation.

8:20 p.m. - Out of room stating "I want to get out of here!" Decreased agitation noted. Talked with mother on the phone and then went back to room. Took halter monitor off. Refused to put it back on.

8/8/89

2:00 p.m. - Have had no observed episodes of agitation on this shift. Patient ambulates with unsteady gait.

5:00 p.m. - Patient in bed. Dinner set up on tray table. Half-way through meal, patient began to sound congested. Lung sounds clear.

5:30 p.m. - Patient remains in room on bed. Patient is calm. No agitated episodes observed. Patient out in hallway. Very unsteady gait noted.

7:30 p.m. - Patient to nurses' desk for phone call from mother. Unable to ambulate due to unsteady gait. Came via wheelchair. Patient stuttering on phone to mother. At times unable to answer her questions. Back to room via wheelchair. To bed with assistance.

8:00 p.m. - Patient ambulated with assist to bathroom to void small amount. Needed three assists to ambulate back to room. Right leg locked. Patient needed assist to move leg.

8:30 p.m. - Resting quietly in bed. Respirations are shallow. Waist support tied to bed.

8:45 p.m. - Talking on phone to mother. Verbalization is slow and broken. Unable to get some words out. Neuroassessment done. Mother upset, says her son may have had a stroke. Told mother that we were not sure of that. Doctor informed per phone of mother's assumptions. Orders received.

9:00 p.m. - Doctor here to see patient and assessment done. More orders received. Mother informed of doctor's presence and orders. Doctor also informed of Sinequan 100

mg. given.
10:30 p.m. - Vitals obtained. Mother informed of patient's
status. Respirations slow and shallow.

During my 8:45 p.m. conversation with Gary, he was
barely able to form words. I could not understand him, no
doubt because of his drugged state. While I was discussing
his status with a nurse, Gary was assisted back to his room.
The nurse told me she received authority to withhold further
medications. But while we were on the phone — before she
was able to communicate the new orders to others — the medication nurse administered more drugs: 100 mg. of Sinequan.
Needless to say, I was wild! No wonder he had slow and shallow respirations and was difficult to awaken the next morning.

8/9/89
11-7 shift - Resting quietly until 3:00 a.m., then found asleep
in wheelchair. Escorted patient back to bed and was very
willing to get back into bed. Tie strap on. Speech slower
and more garbled. Blood pressure 90/60 at 4:00 a.m.
8:20 a.m. - Difficult to awaken patient. When awakened, it
was difficult to keep him awake for breakfast.
9:00 a.m. - Patient requires constant encouragement, cuing, to eat. Eye contact is poor.
9:30 a.m. - Patient is up to shower. He is slow to respond.
Once in shower, he did not assist with any of it. He stares.
12:00 a.m. Patient taken to social area for lunch - He did
not eat well.
1:30 p.m. - Patient has been quite unsteady on his feet
today. Has required wheelchair.
4:00 p.m. - Patient in bed undressed. He would not talk to
caregiver.

8/10/89
11:00 - Found in hall, shoes and slacks off. No stated reason. Re-dressed self with verbal assistance.
11:10 a.m. - Found undressed, shoes and slacks off. States
he was going to bed.
12:30 p.m. - Escorted patient to psychology appointment.
Says he wants to leave Mary Free Bed Hospital and hitch-
hike home.

8/11/89

9:00 a.m. - Spending most of time in room. Very little conversation, most is out of context, i.e., asking nurses age, year of birth.

1:00 p.m. - Resting in bed. Did not speak when spoken to several times.

8/12/89

3:00 a.m. - Patient resting quietly in bed. Side rails up. Call light in reach. Security monitor present on ankle. Holter monitor on.

8:00 a.m. - Patient ate very little for breakfast despite verbal cues to eat. Refused to shave or take a shower.

10:00 a.m. - Patient resting in bed with call light in reach. Patient states he does not believe he is brain injured, though he does believe the present time and location to be correct.

8/13/89

7:00 a.m. - Patient ambulates freely in room and hallway. Patient has poor appetite. Patient refused shower and hygiene tasks, stating "I only shower when I'm dirty."

12:15 p.m. - Patient talks with mother. Staff secures information regarding patient's eating preferences. Patient agrees to take shower per discussion with mother.

5:00 p.m. - With supervision, patient ate in social area. Ate poorly with choking noted.

7:00 p.m. - Patient in social area playing game with staff. Patient abruptly got up and walked away. When asked why, patient stated, "Because you are too easy to beat!"

8:15 p.m. - Patient on phone with mother. Mother on phone states patient wants a milk shake. Milk shake was given, but patient refused it.

8/14/89

9:00 a.m. - Patient is oriented to place and time and calendar date. Patient enjoys removing clothes.

1:30 p.m. - Patient reacts defensively when asked about bowel habits: "I go when I have to go."

4:00 p.m. - Patient in bed with shirt and pants off. Patient oriented to day and time. Patient does not believe he is in a hospital.

9:00 p.m. - Patient remains in bed. Patient does not believe he's brain injured.

8/15/89
8:00 a.m. - Patient eating in social area. Cues needed to eat.
11:30 a.m. - Patient undressed self and put himself to bed. Asked patient why he undressed himself and patient stated he was in bed. Asked why he was in bed. Patient stated he was tired.
1:00-3:00 p.m. - Escorted patient to p.m. appointments.
4:00 p.m. - Patient in room, sitting in bed watching TV. Patient ate supper in social area with parents present. Patient ate well.
8:00 p.m. - Sinequan 25 mg. HELD PER FAMILY REQUEST.

8/16/89
12 a.m. - Patient in hall talking about his age and the year it is now, but is easily directed back to bed. Patient seems more aware tonight.
10:00 a.m. - Shower and shampoo given with minimal assistance. Parents here for final instructions and any problem-solving needed.
11:15 a.m. - Discharged home to parents. Walked out front door.

Without his family around, Gary simply didn't do well. His confusion and frustration sharpened. His behavior — the refusals to eat, the hostile reactions to staff, and the attempts to leave — was a plea for help. He did not know that we were trying to help him. In his mind, he was being held against his will, causing anger and agitation.

The staff at Mary Free Bed were trained to handle brain injury victims. Even so, Gary apparently couldn't be *handled* — at least not without the assistance of drug intervention. While drugs may have slowed him down, rendering him easier to manage, they also compounded his confusion.

The team concluded that Gary was not a candidate for transitional living. Although I was thoroughly disappointed, a part of me was relieved to be taking Gary home. One thing seemed clear: Progress is impossible if Gary resists his environment and medication is required to subdue him.

8

HEART STRINGS

Hope, the patient medicine for disease, disaster, sin.
                                           - Wallace Rice

Big, puffy clouds inched across the sky, sometimes blocking the sun, as we drove north from Grand Rapids. The normal summer road crews were hard at work: shirts off, machines humming, smoke rising from the new blacktop, orange-
vested men funneling two-lane traffic into one.

Gary — legs crossed, his jaw working on a fresh piece of
gum — seemed happy and relaxed; but I was troubled about
what had happened and worried about his future. Superficial
chatter found its way out of my mouth, but my private thoughts
strayed in countless directions. Our one hope to place Gary
in an appropriate setting had now been extinguished; Gary's
brain injury was simply too severe for the transitional living
program.

Since Gary had limited resources, it appeared we were
down to just two options. We could place him in a state institution or convalescent home — but that seemed unworkable.
Or we could create a permanent living arrangement for him at
home; this, we weren't yet ready to accept either. In any case,
discussion of Gary's future living arrangements had to be set
aside. There was a more immediate problem.

Though not accepted for the program, Gary's hospitalization at Mary Free Bed was not in vain. The cardiac work up
and the Holter monitor revealed a serious arrhythmia. We
were informed that Gary had 2400 extra heart beats in a 24-
hour period. Sudden death could be imminent. This serious

condition took precedence over every other consideration.

When we arrived home, I called my husband's cardiologist Dr. Anthony at his Green Bay office. Dr. Anthony advised us to come to Green Bay immediately for extensive testing. So, after a few days in Escanaba, we left for Green Bay, jolted by the notion that Gary would probably have to be hospitalized again.

The two-hour drive from Escanaba to Green Bay gave me time to think. As we made our way southwest from Escanaba toward Menominee, I gazed out across the vast expanse of Lake Michigan. Watching the sun's reflections dance off the water, my mind filled with questions. *What if Gary needed open-heart surgery? Would he survive? Would it rectify the arrhythmia? After all that he has been through, are we going to lose Gary?*

I thought about my college semester starting in a week. *Should I drop out of school?* I had entered college the summer after Gary's heart attack, at age 55 — not with a goal in mind but as a diversion. I concluded that, somehow, another focus would help me keep my sanity. It would take years for me to accept the tragic few moments that changed my son forever, and changed all our lives too.

In class, and while doing assignments, thoughts of Gary flashed like neon signs in my head. I spoke to everyone, instructors and students alike, about my son. I researched brain injury for my writing classes. In speech class, my talks were all about Gary. As time went on, the character of my education became less a diversion, more a pursuit of knowledge — knowledge that could be marshalled to help Gary. I began to concentrate my studies in psychology and social work, constantly seeking out information and resources for Gary's rehabilitation.

We entered Menominee, located about 50 miles southwest along Lake Michigan from Escanaba. Proceeding through town, we drove past the pleasant-looking white house in the center of town, where we had lived for two years. Though Gary Senior and I had grown up in Escanaba and both of our older children graduated from Escanaba High School, varying circumstances had brought us all to Menominee in the mid-

1970s. First our daughter Vicki and her husband Dave settled there, where she worked at our dry cleaning business. Then Gary Senior, Jeff, and I moved there after divesting some of our businesses in Escanaba. Gary and Kris, who had moved to San Diego shortly after their marriage, also decided to settle in Menominee upon returning to the Midwest. We drove over the Menominee River into Marinette, Wisconsin, then southwest another 50 or so miles to Green Bay.

Once in Green Bay, we drove to Bellin Memorial Hospital, where Gary was admitted on August 21, 1989. Dr. Anthony performed a cardiac catheterization, which involved injecting dye into Gary's cardiovascular system to determine the extent of any plaque blockage in his arteries. As with any surgical procedure, there is some risk associated with the test.

As my husband and I nervously waited for the procedure to be completed, my thoughts wandered back to a day in 1975 when I sat here awaiting the outcome of the same procedure — only back then, it was Gary Senior who was in surgery.

At the time, Gary Senior had a cholesterol level over 400. I remembered listening, dazed, as Dr. Anthony explained my husband's test results and prognosis. "Severe, diffuse artery disease. Plaque has built up in the arteries and completely occluded two of them; a third artery is 90 percent occluded. Surgery would be risky."

"How long does he have to live?" I asked, fearing the answer.

"Statistically speaking? From one to five years."

How could this be? My husband was only 44 at the time. Doctor Anthony was, in effect, telling us that we would *not* grow old together. It didn't seem real. Just the evening before, we had a carefree dinner together in a Green Bay restaurant; now, today, my husband was sentenced to death!

Fourteen years later, as we waited for Gary Junior's results, I told my husband — for the first time — of the fears that had engulfed me back in 1975. At the time, I showed only strength and a positive attitude, but this was simply a veneer, a mask for my inner fear and pain. Now, through some bizarre coincidence, here we were again, both together, both awaiting the outcome of the same procedure — this time on our firstborn, Gary.

In one sense, though, it wasn't so bizarre nor even a coincidence. Given the important role heredity plays in heart disease, it was even predictable. His genes tell the story. Not only did Gary's dad have open-heart surgery at 44, but his paternal grandfather had a fatal heart attack at age 53. Two of Gary's great uncles died of heart attacks in their early 50's. My family background was equally compromised. A heart attack took my father at age 33; my brother was 45 when he succumbed to a heart attack after a treadmill test. And my mother, a diabetic, experienced two heart attacks before she died at 73.

Dr. Anthony walked toward us. "He tolerated the procedure well. Gary has severe diffuse artery disease. His right coronary artery is totally occluded."

My husband asked if Gary's case of artery disease was as bad as his own.

"Similar or just as severe," he answered.

Dr. Anthony, a very empathetic and caring person whom we had known for years, looked pained. His eyes were downcast as he answered our questions.

"What are Gary's options?" I asked.

"He would probably be a candidate for heart bypass surgery — or you could do nothing and let nature take its course." With that, Dr. Anthony left the room.

We waited for Gary to be wheeled in from the recovery room.

Let nature take its course? Do nothing? This is our child! How could we do nothing? Was he subtly implying that — in the case of a severely brain-injured man that may be totally dependent upon others for the rest of his life — doing nothing may be the humane thing to do? But to a mother, the natural thing to do was to give him every opportunity to live. There was only one answer. We would meet with the heart surgeon.

Earlier that day, Gary's heart showed signs of irregularity. According to nursing notes, he was experiencing 20 premature ventricular contractions (PVCs) per minute. On one occasion, while sleeping, he had an episode of over 30 PVCs per minute.

That evening, the heart surgeon Dr. Soeter further explained the severe status of Gary's arteries. In addition to the coronary bypass surgery, Dr. Soeter recommended that Gary have a defibrillator patch lead system implanted in his chest. Once in place, a defibrillator can automatically shock the heart if a serious arrhythmia occurs, much like defibrillator paddles are sometimes used in emergencies to shock the heart to get it pumping again.

Dr. Soeter said he would be joined by surgeons from Milwaukee for the implantation procedure. He tried to include Gary in the conversation. Gary listened for a while but then began to interrupt: "How old are you, Doc?" I wasn't sure if he grasped the information and couldn't deal with it, or if he didn't comprehend the seriousness of the procedure.

Gary was discharged, and we left the hospital. We were scheduled to return in three days for the surgery, but the hospital called to delay it for eight more days. Apparently, Dr. Soeter had an emergency surgery, and we would have to wait for the next available date that the Milwaukee surgeons could be present to implant the defibrillator patch lead system.

Meanwhile, I returned to classes at the local community college. I went through the motions, but I wasn't absorbing the lectures. I was consumed instead with the serious matter that lay ahead. I worried about the surgery. Even though school had helped propel me through difficult situations, I began to second-guess my decision to continue.

Then, before we could return to Green Bay for the surgery, Gary had an episode. Physically gasping for air, he complained that he couldn't breathe. We rushed him to the emergency room at St. Francis Hospital near our home in Escanaba. Emotions ran high; he was stabilized but remained in the hospital overnight. Although he survived this episode, I counted the moments until his scheduled surgery. I wanted to rush him to Green Bay before something else happened, yet I was also frightened about the actual surgery. *Will he survive? Are we doing the right thing?*

Within a few days, we left for Green Bay. My husband

and I were apprehensive. Gary, by contrast, was carefree and seemingly detached from what lay ahead. He loved riding in the car. Perhaps he was more fortunate than most cardiac patients. His brain injury spared him the normal anxieties most people experience before a risky surgery.

The Bellin admitting nurse was originally from Escanaba. Gary graduated with her, and we knew her family. That's how it is in a small community; everyone knows something about everyone, some good and some bad. We arrived fraught with tension, but as we exchanged small talk — about mutual acquaintances, our families, her position at Bellin — our tension lessened. She expressed empathy for Gary's tragedy, including his wife's decision to leave him.

I let her know that we preferred Gary's surgery to be a private matter. Being here, going through this with our son was traumatic and difficult. I didn't want any visitors — not even Kris and the boys. Whether that was right or wrong, I can't say. I only know that, with all the stress, I was near a breakdown myself. I needed to reduce potential strife and get through this difficult time.

Gary was escorted to his room.

"Why am I here?" he asked. "I'm not sick!"

"You're here to have heart bypass surgery," I responded.

His mouth opened and his eyes widened.

"*HEART BYPASS SURGERY?*" he exclaimed in disbelief.

But in the next instant, it was back to, "How old am I?" or "What year is it?"

Then, a short time later: "Mom, what am I doing in this hospital?"

Nurses flitted in and out, garnering additional medical history. That evening the anesthesiologist visited to explain the procedure. Gary interrupted with the usual questions about his age and the year. Most of the staff were baffled by Gary's behavior. Although they were professionals, they lacked experience with a brain injured person.

Dr. Soeter came to answer last-minute questions and have Gary sign the consent form. He expressed concern about Gary's ability to grasp the serious nature of the surgery.

"I almost feel as if I'm taking advantage of him," he said.

"Should he be signing a consent form?"

"Gary does not have a guardian," I responded. "Legally, he *can* sign for himself."

With that issue resolved, the doctor continued explaining the actual procedure, time needed, and what to expect afterward.

It was 8:00 p.m. I kissed Gary good-bye and left him and his dad in the room. The game plan was for me to drive the two hours home, attend my morning classes, then return to Green Bay about noon the next day. Gary would be in surgery, so there was nothing I could do.

As I drove home, my eyes clouded with tears, apprehensive about what lay ahead. I slept very little that night. I went to my abnormal psychology class in the morning, but within ten minutes, I approached my instructor and said: "I need to be with my son, who is having heart bypass surgery this morning." I continued explaining the situation through my tears. At that point, I didn't care if I *ever* returned to school!

I drove back to Green Bay, alone with my thoughts. *This very minute my son is lying on a table in the operating room, hooked up to the lung bypass machine, his heart exposed. Maybe he won't survive. I should have been there when they wheeled him into surgery this morning. Isn't that what mothers are all about — being there? How could I have tried to attend school in the middle of this? It was unconscionable. Please God, you've answered so many prayers, just by the fact that Gary is still with us. Don't stop now!*

When I arrived at the hospital, my husband was sitting in the waiting room being comforted by Dr. Soeter's nurse.

I can't explain why feelings of jealousy were mixed with my grief and anxiety. Maybe it was guilt from not being there. Maybe it was pure and simple jealousy that this person — and not I — was comforting my husband!

At first, I ignored her as I impatiently questioned my husband. I'm sure she sensed some of my feelings. She offered to get a progress report from surgery.

When she returned, I had settled down somewhat. She was extremely informative about the implantation of the defibrillator patch lead system. She reported that everything was going well. The bypasses were completed, and the surgeons were working on the implantation of the device. Before long, Dr. Anthony showed his concern, stopping by for a reassuring talk with us.

What seemed like endless hours passed. Even after the surgery was complete, there was a long period before we could see Gary. Finally, Gary was transferred to his room. But problems developed. A nurse assigned to him reported: "He is not awake yet. He's losing blood."

As we entered Gary's room, the visual sight of him — the hissing of the ventilator, tubes taped to his mouth, monitors all around him — brought back uncomfortable memories of seeing him for the first time in Kansas after his cardiac arrest. His head was arched back and he appeared gray, still, and helpless. I stared in disbelief. I felt weak and powerless to do anything. I began to sob. My husband put both hands around my shoulders and led me out of the room. We sat in a private waiting area while the nurses continued their monitoring.

Over the next several hours, Gary's blood loss continued, and several units of blood were ordered. Dr. Soeter made frequent visits throughout the day and into the early evening to check on Gary. When he wasn't present, he remained in constant phone communication with staff on Gary's status.

Gary's surgery was on Thursday. By Sunday evening, the bleeding had lessened and Gary began to stabilize. Later I was told that if the bleeding problem had not been alleviated, another surgery would have been necessary.

Then, by Monday, Gary amazed the staff and doctors. He was fully conscious, perpetually in motion, talkative, and in high spirits. His memory seemed better for short periods, but he had no memory of undergoing heart surgery.

The defibrillator was implanted, but it was not connected because Gary's severe arrhythmia had been alleviated as a result of the bypass surgery. Nonetheless, it was in place and would require only minor surgery should it ever have to be activated.

After Monday, Gary's recuperation was swift. I wondered if the mind does play a part in healing. Gary didn't remember the surgery; therefore, he behaved as if he never had it. His cardiac recuperative powers were truly profound.

Once at home, I resumed classes. Within a couple of days, Gary's son Arlo called. I informed him of the surgery. Kris and the boys came over to take Gary for a ride. When they brought him back, Arlo escorted his dad to the door. He noted how thin Gary now appeared. The combination of those weeks at Mary Free Bed Hospital and the heart surgery had taken its toll.

By mid-September, the high school across the street from our house was again bustling with activity. Just weeks before, when we had transported Gary for his surgery, the high school grounds were quiet, the doors were shuttered, and only one car was visible in the parking lot. Now, the lot was almost full, and from our living room window we could see the football team and school band practicing. Bright-colored autumn leaves had begun to appear on the trees, signaling the change of season. The sun warmed the crisp, cool air.

As I gazed out the window, I was interrupted by the phone ringing. My sister Pauline's friend was on the other end. "Are you aware that Pauline has been diagnosed with a rare fatal illness?" she asked. "Pauline knew your hands were full with your son's surgery and care, so she chose not to tell you."

Saddened by this unexpected news, I called Pauline at the country club where she worked. She nonchalantly explained that her bone marrow was becoming fibrous, affecting her blood production. She didn't seem that concerned. When I hung up, I thought: *It can't be fatal, not with her attitude.*

But, later, her daughter informed me that Pauline had less than six months to live. A few years earlier, my brother had died at 45 due to a heart problem. Now my only sister was sentenced to die at 51. *Will this nightmare never end?*

Around that time, I found a large cardboard box outside our front door. I began to open it, and became puzzled. Inside the box, clothes and shoes were piled neatly. Then, it dawned on me. *These are Gary's belongings!* Apparently, Kris and the boys had left them. As I searched through his things, I felt sorrowful. Was this his legacy from 15 years of marriage? A box of old clothes discarded on his parents' doorstep? How sad for Gary.

Preempted by the twin ordeals of Mary Free Bed and Gary's heart surgery, my husband and I had not yet discussed Gary's future. To me, however, that box was simply another sign that, yes, Gary was home for good.

The winds of change were still blowing. Nonetheless, it seemed time to settle in and move on with our lives.

9

MOVING ON

Under all skies, all weathers,
man's happiness lies always elsewhere.
- Giacomo Leopardi

September waned before I realized that Gary's family had ceased calling or picking up Gary for visits. Later, I learned Kris and the boys had moved to another state. They did not leave us a forwarding address.

Although Gary's permanent living arrangements were never actually discussed, my husband decided to sell our dry cleaning business. Demands on us were heavy: Gary Senior's failing health, Gary Junior's ongoing care, and my commitment to continuing my education.

Attending college continued to be a great experience for me. I mingled with young people, acted in a theater production, and relished the day-to-day activities that allowed me to lose myself in an entirely different world from what I faced at home.

Jeff and Peggy came home for Christmas 1989. They were expecting their first baby in March.

I helped Gary pick out gifts for Kris and the boys. He made his own choices: sports clothing for the boys and a warm white fur hat with matching gloves for Kris.

Kris and the boys visited her family at Christmas time. They spent a few hours with Gary. I still had not been officially informed of where they lived, although I heard they were in Minnesota.

My sister Pauline spent Christmas with us. It was heartbreaking. She didn't look well at all. With huge dark circles under her eyes, she joked and laughed as though nothing had changed. What a unique woman. She planned a late-January trip to the Bahamas with her daughter and a friend, but she never lived to see the beautiful beaches. Pauline died on January 17, 1990. I will miss her the rest of my life. The country club she managed named a lake after her: Lake Pauline, a tribute to a great woman.

Jeff and Peggy's baby arrived in March 1990. They named her Mary Patricia — *Mary* after Peggy's mother, *Patricia* after me. She goes by Mary Pat.

In the spring, my husband and Gary attended my graduation from the local community college. "I'm proud of you, Mom," Gary said. I beamed, not because of the accomplishment, but because of the appropriateness of his statement. Normal reactions *did* penetrate his confusion on rare occasions.

Those days hold many memories for me, some fond, some terrible. We were light-hearted, or we despaired. We were optimistic, or we felt overwhelmed. For the most part, however, we were dysfunctional. Nothing seemed normal. Every day, over and over, Gary lamented, "I've lost my wife. I've lost my job. I've lost everything." Moreover, my husband and I began to feel the strains of Gary's day-to-day care. Because Gary had no short-term memory, he needed constant cues and encouragement to complete everyday routines that most of us perform effortlessly.

Gary's typical day began with an early morning shower. He needed to be cued to take off his pajamas and underpants; Gary Senior or I would draw his water, place shampoo in his hand, encourage him to wash himself, and often ended up physically washing his backside for him. Then, we'd dry him off and give him underpants to put on. We put the toothpaste in his hand, turned on the water, encouraged him to brush, shut off the water, and then flossed his teeth. We'd set up his electric razor, put it in his hand, and stay there to cue him to assure that he didn't leave the room before the job was done and the razor turned off.

Then came dressing. Gary needed someone to select appropriate clothing and needed constant cuing on each component of the dressing process: Put this on. Button this up. Remove this. Without cues, he would go back to bed or leave the room undressed or only half dressed. For breakfast, as with all meals, the food had to be prepared, then sufficiently cut up to make it easy for him to swallow. Since he tried to talk while eating, he needed close monitoring to prevent choking. Almost every bite had to be encouraged. Sometimes I simply had to feed him like a baby to maintain good nutrition and health.

All traffic patterns in the house had to be kept open and free of clutter or Gary would stumble. Cleaning the bathroom was a never-ending process because of his inattention to what he is doing. Likewise, laundry always seemed to be piling up.

We'd take him to medical appointments for evaluations as needed, including pulmonary function tests, blood work, and CAT scans. We cleaned his ears and cut his nose hairs. A haircut was a major undertaking; he constantly moved his head, touched the stylist, and perseverated on the year and everyone's age. And every three months, we took Gary to a podiatrist for clipping, grooming and nail fungus check.

As appropriate, I would also work with Gary on exercises for his drooping shoulder and stooped posture. In the cognitive area, we'd work on spelling, math, and general reasoning. Throughout the day, we also needed to monitor Gary for signs that he needs to urinate or have a bowel movement.

All of this left us feeling exhausted at night. Gary Senior and I would want to sleep. But, Gary sometimes wandered at night. Before we began to lock our bedroom door at night, Gary — perhaps several times during the night — would hover over our bedside and demand answers to the same questions on which he perseverated all day: "How old am I? What year is it? Why am I here?" Or sometimes, we would hear the door slam in the wee hours of the morning. My husband would jump from bed to find Gary outside in his underwear checking the license plates in order to find out the year: winter or summer, it didn't matter.

Other times, we'd hear him opening kitchen drawers, shuffling through papers or mail, and checking the contents of boxes. Attempting to uncover the source of his confusion and a possible key to recovery, Gary had become a detective in the night. He was on a covert mission with an objective that seemed even more more important than national security — finding out what *really* happened to him.

Clearly, Gary needed more than this daily routine. He needed more structure in his life, occupation to absorb his energy. Yet the laborious daily routine and lack of sleep left Gary Senior and me feeling exhausted even before our day began. We practically dreaded each morning. So, I began searching for help locally.

Eventually, Michigan Rehabilitation Services helped place Gary in a work program for the mentally retarded. It was the only program available in Escanaba. At the work site, Gary and the others painted wooden stakes for the state highway department. Three days a week, a bus would transport him to and from our home to the work site. One morning, sun shining, Gary was in our front yard seeming to enjoy the day. Gary waved at the bus as it rumbled down the street toward our house. The bus driver recognized Gary and stopped in front as he had done on previous days. Although it wasn't a work day for him, Gary climbed into the bus and was transported off to the work site. We didn't know where he was until we received a call from a representative of the work program informing us that Gary showed up for work on his day off.

While this program seemed to be a good idea, ultimately it didn't work out. Gary needed one-on-one attention, but the work program operated on a six-to-one ratio. Gary didn't stay on task and continually asked, "Why am I with these retarded people? I'm not retarded."

Gary perceived that he didn't belong there. After all, here is a man who can play chess (though after several moves, his weakened concentrational skills cause him to abort the game), pass a state driver's test with flying colors, and perform other important cognitive deeds — at least for brief periods. Here is a man whose short-term memory and other deficits prevent him from executing certain tasks, but whose cognitive function is quite capable for the moment. Here is a man whose long-term memory is largely intact, who is able to remember how he used to be. Even though brain injured, he is still able to make comparisons. And when he saw himself teamed up with mentally retarded people, his self esteem suffered — it simply didn't fit his image of how the *old* Gary would have spent his time.

Meanwhile, I was at a decision-point in my education. After completing the two-year associate degree program at the local community college in Escanaba, the University of Michigan offered me a generous scholarship. Located in Ann Arbor, the main campus is about an eight-hour drive into southern Michigan. I vacillated on the question of whether to continue my education — there or anywhere else. But, with encouragement from my husband, we left for Ann Arbor to learn more about the school's social work curriculum and to check out therapy and other programs for people with a brain injury.

We stayed in a hotel near campus and spent an absolutely horrid night. Gary was up all night, sometimes wandering out in the hall in his underwear. He acted out inappropriately when we were in restaurants. The lack of structure and the change of locale overwhelmed him, and his response to this stress overwhelmed us. It seemed a pretty strong omen against transferring to the University of Michigan.

I decided, instead, to continue my education at Northern Michigan University in Marquette, about an hour drive north from Escanaba. They offered a bachelor's degree in social work, and I was determined to pursue it.

About six weeks before the fall 1990 semester began, we went to Marquette to secure an apartment through student housing. Upon completion of the application, the clerk informed me that certain documents, including our marriage license, would be necessary to process the application.

"We've been married forty years — are you serious?" I said in disbelief.

"I realize that, but our rules require proof of marriage from any student occupying family housing."

We laughed about it afterward. We felt like a couple of kids anticipating life on campus. We shopped for a cheap toaster, a coffeemaker, a couple of throw rugs — the usual items needed to set up light housekeeping. I enrolled full-time; my husband, part-time.

Just before classes began, we moved into a one-bedroom apartment. To promote a stable environment, we gave the bedroom to Gary, and we slept on a pull-out sofa in the living room. We planned to spend weekends at our home in Escanaba.

Once again, we were caught up in a cycle of change, sometimes wonderful, sometimes excruciating, with Gary ever at the center. My husband, a history buff, had mixed emotions about attending school again at age 60. He enjoyed the history classes, but was angered — even threatened — by some attitudes and viewpoints of the young students, many of whom identified with the young, liberal-minded instructors.

Gary Senior, a conservative patriot from the World War II era, was bothered by the revisionist ideas that surfaced in his political science class. He complained that the professor constantly criticized the U.S. role in history, its presidents, and its foreign policy. The instructor, he said, had an ardent "blame-America-first" philosophy. More often than not, Gary Senior came home frustrated. After a while, perhaps as a way of dealing with the frustration, he began to joke about it. He lamented that the instructor didn't *even* like the Green Bay Packers, as if that was some kind of final litmus test, a confirmation that there was *indeed* something improper — perhaps even sinister — about the class.

At times he also felt conspicuous because of his age. He was older than all the teachers. He searched for other gray-haired individuals and finally discovered that there were at least two other students from his generation.

In one of his classes, each student was assigned to look up some significant news item that had been reported on his or her birth date. My husband found a newspaper article, dated March 28, 1931, announcing that the State of Michigan would soon require a driver's license to operate an automobile — quite a contrast from astronauts landing on the moon! This really did make him feel like a relic compared to the other students.

Overall, however, the educational experience was enjoyable for both of us. Test days were met with anxiety, but we were usually rewarded for being well-prepared.

Meanwhile, Gary didn't fare so well from the changes. Every Monday morning we drove back to classes in Marquette. Gary would question us repeatedly: "Where are we going?" "Why are we going there?" When we arrived at our apartment, he accused us of setting up the apartment for him so we could "get rid of" him. No amount of reassurance would console him.

We scheduled our classes so one of us was always with Gary. I was still searching for a meaningful program, one that would give Gary structure. I made an appointment with the Community Mental Health office in Marquette. It took weeks to get an appointment, but I waited. I waited while Gary's records were gathered from all the different hospitals. Then, I waited for a follow-up call.

Finally, I received the call:

"Hello, Mrs. Abrahamson," he said. "The occupational therapist and myself work twice a week with a small group of boys who have brain injuries. The outings are community-type activities — lunch in the park, bowling, or shopping. The boys have a voice in their preference of activities. After reviewing Gary's records, we would like to include Gary in the group."

"Great!" I replied. "Gary needs new experiences and opportunities to make outside friends."

I welcomed the respite when Gary went on group outings. I could study without interruptions. When Gary was around, I had to struggle with double tracking: studying on one track, while answering Gary's perseverative questions on another.

Once in a while, I'd answer wrong. When he'd ask "How old am I?" I would unconsciously reply with my own age: "58." He really *did* know the right answers because he would shriek, "I'm not 58, you are!" Or again, listening with one ear, I would mistakenly tell him I was 40. He'd shriek in response, "You're not 40, I am!"

It wasn't long before Gary's perseverative questions began to unnerve some of the boys in the group. In fact, he was so disruptive — for example, yelling if he didn't get a response or the right answer — that the case manager phoned me and, in an apologetic tone, said, "For the benefit of the other boys,

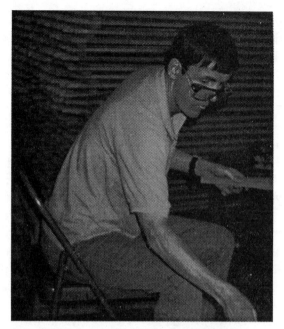

As part of a sheltered workshop, Gary makes
highway stakes for the State of Michigan, 1990.

Gary's pay stubs. He was paid by the piece and didn't make a lot.

we are going to have to drop Gary from the group." I understood why immediately.

While we pursued our schooling, Gary became fixated on work. He repeatedly said, "I need a job. I need to work!" It's almost as if he thought his life would return to "normal" if only he had a job. Imagine — especially for a man, a breadwinner — what a huge part of a person's existence and identity is caught up in a job, one's ability to provide security. No wonder Gary was obsessed with the word "work" and with its meaning.

I talked to the case manager about Gary's work obsession. Given Gary's fixation on it, we both agreed that another trial work period was in order.

The case manager selected a sheltered workshop with mentally retarded individuals. The job involved wood-working, stamping and making highway stakes for the State of Michigan.

A bus picked up Gary three days a week at 8:00 a.m. We scurried to complete the shower-shave-and-breakfast routine. Gary was tired but eager. I packed his lunch and his dad waited outside with Gary in the sub-zero cold weather until the bus arrived.

One week, my social work class scheduled a field trip to Gary's work site. Although I had visited the site before Gary started the work program, I was eager to view Gary at work without his knowledge.

He was so pathetic, so sad. He appeared bewildered. The bell rang for break time. Gary looked confused as everyone proceeded to the lunchroom. I entered the lunchroom and made my presence known to Gary.

"Where's your lunch, Gary?" I asked.

"I'm eating it" chirped a young handicapped person next to Gary.

Poor Gary. He was hungry, but didn't recall bringing a lunch, let alone knowing which lunch was his. He looked as if someone had hammered him on the head. Confused and dazed, he asked, "Why am I here? I want to go home!" Both the work site director and I agreed that, for Gary, this was not the right direction at this time.

When I took Gary home, he wanted to lie down in his bed; though it was still early afternoon, he seemed exhausted. I still had some time before my next class, so I sat down at the kitchen table with a stack of papers — hospital records, progress reports from physicians and neuropsychologists, letters to congressmen and agencies, notes about possible programs and therapies — and began contemplating our next step.

Groping through the sheaf of papers, I came across this letter. Gary penned it just 15 days before his cardiac arrest.

Saturday, October 10, 1987

Dear Mom and Dad,

Thank you so much for the nice card and thoughts for my birthday. I also thank you for the money you sent me. That is always something I can use and always comes in the right size and color. I bought some nursing uniforms with it. Every time I turn around, I am needing extra money since starting this program. It will all be worth it some day. I am real anxious to start my clinical rotation next week in obstetrics. I hope to specialize in some area of nursing such as drug and alcohol rehabilitation or psychiatric nursing. We have a state mental institution about 20 miles away that is crying for registered nurses and start them at about $25,000 a year. Another possibility for me, which I think would be extremely interesting, is a nurse anesthetist. At our Great Bend hospital, we have one anesthesiologist and five nurse anesthetists. The anesthesiologist oversees the nurses. These nurses make about $40,000 here. They also have good benefits. I would need a bachelor's degree and one year of nurse anesthetist school which would give me a master's degree in nursing. I am doing well in my classes this semester — A's and B's. I got the first C I have ever gotten on a nursing exam last month, and it bothered me for a week afterwards. I could hardly sleep the night I found out. I can remember when I got a C in high school, I was thrilled. Times and people change, I guess.

Arlo has been doing real well on the 9th grade football team — kicker and tight end. He wears glasses now and

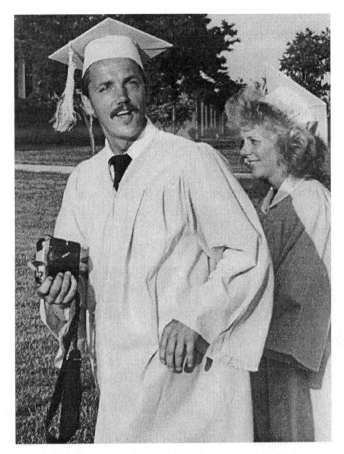

Gary graduates from college — plans more education to become a nurse anesthetist, 1987.

looks real good in them, although they do make him look older.

Leif Eric was in the area-wide pass, punt, and kick competition last Saturday, and took 1st place in the 8-year-old division. He won a very nice plaque and must return for district competition next week. We are quite proud of him.

Say hello to grandma for us and tell her we are thinking of her and praying for her to get better. I know it must be hard on you to watch her deteriorate that way. I guess you just have to keep your head up and do what you can for her and know that she is in God's hands.

I got a phone call from Jeff the night of my birthday. It

was really nice to hear from him. Kris talked with Peggy for quite a while also. Kris said although they have never met, she thinks they would become very good friends if they lived close by. I sent a card and letter off to Jeff after I talked on the phone with him to tell how proud of him I am. He really has a lot going for him. Well, we'll wrap this up for now. Thanks again for the card and money. Write when you can as we all enjoy hearing from you.

Love,   Gary

P.S. Enclosed is a graduation picture with the president of the college.

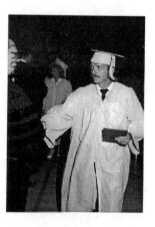

In the months following Gary's cardiac arrest, I read this letter countless times. I had not yet answered it when the tragedy occurred; for a while, I punished myself for that.

10

LIFE STRUGGLES

Once one determines that he or she has a mission in life,
that it's not going to be accomplished without a great deal of pain,
and that the rewards in the end may not outweigh the pain
... then when it comes, you survive it.
- Richard Nixon

The fall semester at Northern Michigan University was a novel experience for us all. Following each frustration or disappointment, there came a delightful or inspirational event to even the score.

But there were risks. The twin pillars of familiarity and structure were important for Gary's well-being; yet this experience was unfamiliar, a venture into unchartered waters. Juggling class schedules, looking after Gary, and trying to find study-time was a persistent struggle. We began optimistically, but by mid-October I had my doubts. Perhaps our dual existence — four days on campus in Marquette and weekends at our home in Escanaba — was a contributing problem. But whatever the cause, Gary's frustration increased.

Again, just like before, Gary vented most of his frustration toward Gary Senior.

"Dad, how old am I? What year is this?"

His dad answered correctly, but Gary shot back:

"Oh, you're full of shit, aren't you?"

Then, ten seconds later:

"How come you let this happen to me, Dad?"

Five seconds after that:

"Why do I have to go through this bullshit? *Why?*"

Another five seconds: "You don't care about me, do you,

Dad?"

Ten seconds later: "I'm lost — too bad, huh?"

This would go on for hours, as if Gary was purposely try-ing to start fights with his dad. Gary Senior called it "Chinese water torture," sort of like tying someone up and letting water drip in the same place on his head for a long period. Each individual drop, by itself, is harmless; it's the repetition that creates the torture.

I pondered why. In the deep recesses of Gary's psyche could be found — perhaps — a reason for this intermittent antagonism toward his dad. Maybe it was something that had been subconscious, suppressed, or dormant until the brain injury ravaged his inhibitions and helped expose it. I went all the way back to Gary's infancy searching for answers.

Gary was always demanding. Even his screaming was different from most babies. As he learned to walk and talk, Gary's demanding nature soon translated into defiance. I spanked him, but it didn't help, and I became frustrated car-ing for him. About one year later, his sister Vicki was born. She was Gary's opposite. While he demanded more than his share of attention, she was passive. His assertiveness and her passiveness were manifest in even the most basic daily routines. After giving them each a bottle of milk, I would have to watch closely because Gary would drink his, throw it to the side, then take hers. He took it even if he didn't drink it all, and she would sit by passively — no cries, no warning that she wasn't getting nourishment. Gary gained weight for both of them until I realized what was going on. We were young parents. In some ways, I don't believe we provided enough boundaries for Gary.

But, when he grew older, my husband disciplined him with a belt. I, too, must take responsibility for threatening delayed punishment. It was the old cliche: "Wait 'til your father gets home." Yet, watching my husband take off his belt even frightened me. My husband became frustrated by the situation. His father was a strict disciplinarian, and the mere threat of punishment was enough to deter a young Gary Se-nior. He couldn't understand why Gary Junior wasn't afraid of punishment.

Knowledge from social work classes reinforced my grow-

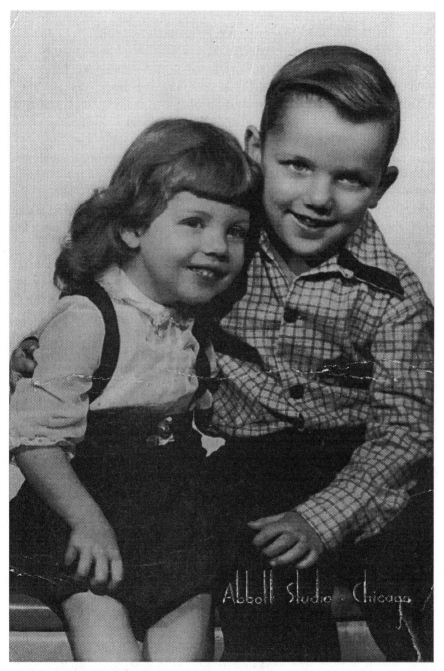

Gary and sister Vicki as children, 1953

ing belief that Gary's current behavior could, at least in part, be traced to his upbringing. Gary's distaste of any authority — whether parents, educators, or peers — was probably hatched in our strict home environment. Perhaps in today's society, belt spanking would be considered abusive. But as young parents, we just wanted the best for Gary. We thought we were doing what was needed to mold him to be a good boy and responsible citizen.

Unfortunately, after his cardiac arrest, Gary's general resistance to authority actually impeded his ability to benefit from certain therapies. Moreover, therapists unintentionally added to the problem by adopting treatment styles too rigid for Gary's resistive personality. What works for one individual with a brain injury may not work for another.

Whatever the cause of Gary's underlying hostility toward his father, it was unsettling. Looking for inner meaning, we began to wonder whether this was some sort of divine retribution for our mistakes as young parents. In any case, the disruptions occurred daily. And, divinely inspired or not, it increased my stress.

Endlessly, I worried. *When will the next altercation occur? Will it escalate out of control?* The turmoil affected our marriage. There were days when my husband and I didn't speak to each other at all.

Now, in addition to our responsibility of caring for Gary, we endured that responsibility under increasingly hostile conditions. Gary Senior began to crack. He spoke darkly of "getting out of this situation." He even began to talk of suicide.

"Maybe we'd all be better off dead," he said. "This isn't living; in fact, it may even be a kind of hell."

Silently I watched our marriage disintegrate. I was consumed only with Gary's needs. About this time, Jeff was in Chicago on a business trip. He picked up Vicki at her home north of Milwaukee and met us at a restaurant in Menominee, Michigan. We talked and searched for solutions. "Dad, maybe you should spend a couple of weeks with me?" Vicki offered. We felt their concern and sympathy, but they couldn't offer more than Band-Aid treatment for a situation that seemed now to require major surgery.

Desperate, I called the Community Mental Health office

in Escanaba. We went to the office for a meeting, where I explained our needs.

"*We* need help," I said. Even a respite away from Gary for a couple hours daily might give us the breathing room we needed. The options were limited, however. In Escanaba, no programs existed for people with brain injuries; and Gary had already tried the sheltered workshop for the mentally retarded, but that didn't work — partly because it offended Gary's false pride to be placed among those whose disablement could be observed physically. By contrast, we reasoned, mental illness does not usually take on outward physical manifestations; so, we asked Community Mental Health whether Gary could be placed in the partial day program for the mentally ill.

Gary Senior needed help also. At a minimum, Gary Senior's hints of suicide were a desperate call for help. Counseling certainly seemed to be in order.

Finally, *Gary* needed help. He needed speech, occupational, physical, and cognitive therapies to help rehabilitate him.

The Community Mental Health staff seemed sympathetic and promised another meeting in order to present us with whatever services could be provided. Meanwhile, we fought off the urge to take any hasty steps, and went on with our lives as best we could.

About that time, Michigan Rehabilitation Services requested a new neuropsychological evaluation for Gary. We arranged to have Gary tested in Green Bay during our Thanksgiving vacation from classes. The evaluation included this entry.

Summing up today's test results, it appears that only slight insignificant improvements have been made in Mr. Abrahamson's overall cognitive functioning level in the past two years, and he remains severely impaired in terms of memory functioning, executive capabilities, and complex problem solving skills. Verbal intelligence has shown the best improvement, but again the gains are far from robust. Visuospatial capabilities and concentration skills continue to appear moderately impaired, though there have been some slight improvements in these areas. Behaviorally, Mr. Abrahamson continues to be somewhat defensive and seems to put people on guard, and his behavior is not appropriate; he perseveratively asks the same series of questions over and over again. Mr. Abrahamson continues to lack complete awareness of his deficits and denied any problems in memory, thinking, or concentration in today's testing.

It has now been over three years since Mr. Abrahamson's [oxygen loss due to heart failure], and the lack of significant improvement in his cognitive functioning suggests that these neuropsychological impairments are likely of a chronic, permanent character. Prognosis for future cognitive improvement, at least of any significance, would unfortunately appear poor.

I discussed these results in detail with Mr. Abrahamson's mother following the evaluation. I told her that, in my opinion, a realistic approach to her son's unfortunate situation is necessary. We discussed that Mr. Abrahamson's cognitive problems are not simply in terms of memory functioning, but that they also extend into the verbal, intellectual, visuospatial, executive, and concentration domains. We also discussed significant concerns related to his behavioral problems.

I recommend that serious consideration be given to placing Mr. Abrahamson in a structured, residential facility geared toward dealing with individuals with brain injury concerns. Certainly, sheltered employment should also be promoted, though obviously, this is a complicated undertaking given Mr. Abrahamson's cognitive and behavioral levels of functioning.

I generally read and analyze each new medical evaluation with a slightly skewed perspective, focusing on any documented gains, even the minuscule ones. Moreover, as Gary's primary caretaker, I was able to recognize gains in Gary that were not documented by the clinicians. Not all gains are subject to measurement by the usual techniques of having Gary draw block designs, assemble puzzles, or recall what he read a half hour ago. Certain subtle improvements are recognizable only by the people who live with the person 24 hours a day, seven days a week, 52 weeks a year.

I know now that these small gains, even if they continue, are not in the aggregate likely to translate into independence for Gary. That said, however, I cannot afford to develop a defeatist attitude. I need to relish each small accomplishment — for both Gary and myself. We just can't give up trying to rehabilitate him.

To avoid triggering false hopes or expectations, clinicians tend to downplay the small improvements. However, this guarded approach — if taken too far — may unnecessarily discourage the victim's caretakers. Clinicians need to be sensitive to this and, if necessary, take a more holistic approach; a more holistic approach recognizes that families need to hear even the smallest good news to offset the overwhelming burden they face; a more holistic approach gives adequate emphasis to the psychological ingredient of good doctoring.

Child psychologists suggest that we should temper constructive criticism with occasional praise. I, for one, am not afraid to admit that — at least when it comes to motivation — adults are perfectly capable of behaving like children!

Christmas 1990 neared. Student housing called.

"Your name has come up for the two-bedroom townhouse you requested," the voice said. "Are you still interested?"

"Still interested?" I replied. "We're elated!"

"We have some painting to complete," she explained. "But you can move in upon your return to school in January."

Surely, we thought, this would make a difference for all of us. Gary would have more freedom to roam. Gary Senior and I would have a real bed.

But when we returned to classes after the holidays, Gary seemed just as troubled, just as paranoid. Again, he thought the new apartment was set up for him — that we were going to leave him there. Apparently, the physical changes in his environment were causing him distress. Many times at night he would come into our room and exclaim in a panicked voice, "Dad, come quick, the moon is falling!" On those occasions, we would get up, reassure him, and comfort him until he went back to sleep.

I was still looking for help and direction regarding the best way to handle Gary, to rehabilitate him, and to make his life more meaningful. I arranged for more evaluations at Marquette General Hospital. Perhaps now, I thought, Gary would be more receptive to speech and occupational therapy. But, again, testing in a clinical hospital setting intimidated Gary, causing him to become agitated. The hospital didn't think he was a good candidate for their therapy programs.

Later, at a brain injury support group meeting, I met a psychologist who was willing to help Gary in her home office. The sessions seemed to go well. I was convinced his progress with her was directly related to the fact that it was one-on-one, in a home environment rather than a hospital. Amazingly, he was able to spend up to three hours with her without becoming seriously agitated.

A special community bus transported Gary to and from these sessions. Michigan Rehabilitation Services funded the therapy and the busing.

One blustery, freezing day, Gary didn't return home on the bus at the usual time. I waited for him, watching out the window, just as a mother might watch for her five-year-old to return from kindergarten. An hour passed. I called the psychologist.

"Gary left on the bus over an hour ago," she said. "I personally put him on the bus."

My mind began to race: *Where could he be?* The bus company was in the business of transporting handicapped people under contract with Michigan Rehabilitative Services. They were well aware of Gary's handicap.

I dialed the bus company.

"We don't know what could have happened to him," said a bus company representative. "We will contact the driver of that bus and report back to you."

Another half hour passed. A Northern Michigan winter has its share of below-zero temperatures. This day was typical — very cold, and the wind, which made it even colder, cut like a knife. *Where is my son?*

Finally, the bus company called back.

"The driver didn't realize you had moved from the apartment into the townhouse after the holidays," she explained.

"The driver remembered dropping Gary off at your old apartment back when Gary was in the work program, so that's where she left him."

Given the severe weather, I was immediately frightened for Gary's life: *My God, he won't know what to do if he goes to the door of the old apartment! He won't even be able to explain his situation to anyone.*

My husband was out the door like a cannon shot. He went to the old apartment — no sign of Gary, nor had anyone seen him. My husband searched frantically while I stayed home in case Gary returned. Moments seemed like hours. *Was Gary a victim of foul play?*

Two hours passed. Suddenly, my husband entered the drive. Gary was with him. Relief overwhelmed all my other emotions.

My husband found Gary about a mile down the road. After he left the bus, Gary apparently walked several blocks and was heading toward a wooded area when my husband spotted him. We shuddered to think what might have happened. He could have stumbled over a rock or a protruding root and lay there, confused, until he froze to death.

Gary had trouble speaking — he could barely move his mouth. His hands, feet, and ears were cold as ice. He shivered for hours and was enraged with us for allowing this to happen. Even today, despite his impaired short-term memory, he can still recall this dreadful day if cued.

I can only imagine his bewilderment as he ambled down the snow-covered street: trudging footsteps, howling wind, hands, feet, and ears growing colder with each step, no clear idea where he was going, forgetting where he came from. Since Gary hadn't grown up in Marquette, the town was unfamiliar to him; he held no long-term memories upon which he could draw to help guide his path. For a dangerous few hours, he was lost in time and space — frozen space.

Soon thereafter — in the middle of the winter semester — we dropped out of school and returned home to Escanaba. My pursuit of a social work degree was put on the back burner.

11

BLOOD, SWEAT AND TEARS

Thy fate is the common fate of all;
into each life some rain must fall.
                    - Henry Wadsworth Longfellow

Gary seemed more content and relaxed when we first arrived home in Escanaba. Although frustration was still evident, he was more manageable.

I continued searching for a structured program to help
him as well as to give us a break. Now that I was out of school,
I had more time. Already, we had done a number of things
aimed at addressing Gary's cognitive and physical needs. There
had been ongoing medical evaluations, heart surgery, attempted placement in a transitional living program, sheltered
workshops; we contacted members of Congress, the Department of Social Services, Michigan Rehabilitation Services, and
the Community Mental Health offices in both Marquette and
Escanaba. Yet, Gary still had unmet needs — and so did we!
Moreover, I seemed to be running out of answers.

I became increasingly impatient at the apparent inaction
of the local Community Mental Health office. While Gary Senior determined that he didn't need or want counseling after
all, we were still playing the waiting game for them to tell us
what, if anything, they could do to place Gary in a partial day
program for the mentally ill. Due apparently to some bureaucratic buck-passing, we went several weeks without being offered anything for Gary, so I decided to seek services elsewhere.

Michigan Rehabilitation Services paid for a computer for
Gary, along with programs recommended by the speech thera-

pist at Marquette General Hospital. I hired a computer-literate individual to work with Gary an hour each day and soon saw slight improvement in his ability to concentrate. However good that hour was for him, however, there are many hours in a day. And during many of them, Gary paced like a caged tiger. He needed additional outlets for his energy. *Perhaps this restlessness is a sign of progress,* I thought. But it certainly wasn't normal to walk from one room to another with nothing meaningful to do.

The month before we left school, I had applied for a promising program through the Social Security Administration. If approved, the PASS Program (Plan to Achieve Self-Support), as it is called, would provide one-on-one direction for Gary while it gave Gary Senior and me a much-needed respite. In February 1991, the agency called to inform me that they had approved the plan I presented to them.

"Yey! The plan's been approved!" I told my husband excitedly. "We're going to get some help." With that news, I called Community Mental Health and told them to close our file: "I will be hiring my own aides for Gary. I can't wait any longer for your help. We need help now."

In short, the PASS program allowed us to hire someone to work with Gary for five hours daily. Under the plan I presented to the agency, this person would assist Gary in pursuit of the most basic social, recreational, and physical activities to help him develop skills to reenter society: shopping for groceries and birthday presents, a picnic in the park, exercise, attending sports events, playing bingo, pool, and miniature golf.

The first person I hired was a recent college graduate with a degree in psychology. Even though we only paid minimum wage since that was all we could afford, she welcomed the opportunity to gain experience in her field.

It changed our lives and Gary's. Five hours a day, Gary was involved in basic, but meaningful, activities. Five hours a day, Gary had someone's undivided attention. Five hours a day, Gary became a part of the community. And five hours a day, my husband and I had respite time away from Gary — thus making the time we *did* spend with him more meaningful and worthwhile; the family dynamic vastly improved.

Over time, help came and went: some left for better jobs, others couldn't handle the intense, sometimes intimidating one-on-one interaction with Gary. I found that the aide's personality was extremely important. Some lacked the skills, patience, or empathy that Gary needed.

Through trial and error, I became better at hiring and training people. I was, it seemed, blazing a trail in a health care wilderness that lacked resources and appropriate programs for those with brain injuries and their families; and whatever programs *were* available were not *readily* available, forcing me to shout aloud in a community that at first couldn't hear — or seemed to ignore — my pleas for help.

I soon discovered that Gary worked better with women than with men. Gary seemed more disturbed, more threatened by taking direction from a man; perhaps he viewed men primarily as competitors — for jobs, for the attention of women, for respect among other men. Women, by contrast, were the object of the competition and a refuge from it. Perhaps taking direction from a man simply reminded him that he was no longer the strong man he perceived himself to be. Whatever the reason, with a woman, his ego was better protected.

This simple program was a godsend. Within weeks, my husband's mental health improved; and under the new circumstances, I began to consider continuing my work toward a bachelor's degree. This time, however, we would not move Gary out of our home environment. If I were to continue, I would commute between Escanaba and Northern Michigan University in Marquette, a 130-mile round-trip. By April, I decided to make that commute and return to school for the summer semester.

In May 1991, just before I returned to school, my son Jeff received a Master's Degree in Business Administration (MBA) from George Washington University in Washington, D.C. My daughter Vicki cared for Gary so we could attend Jeff's graduation. Gary had been with us for two years now. For two years, our primary focus was on him and on the tragedy that had totally engulfed our life. It was good for us to attend Jeff's graduation and bask in his accomplishments.

Meanwhile, we anticipated the usual summer visit from Glenn and Alexis. By letter, they had informed us that they were expecting a child in September. I was especially anxious for their extended visit because their infrequent presence placed them in an objective position to recognize progression or — for that matter — regression in Gary.

Glenn was a cut-up and drew hearty laughter from Gary. When Glenn was around, Gary's demeanor — in terms of body language and facial expressions — came the closest to matching his pre-trauma demeanor. In fact, Gary would break out in a smile at the mere sight of Glenn approaching the house, perhaps in anticipation of what was to come. Since Gary's long-term memory was largely intact, he had no problem recalling the good times and laughter they had shared in the past. It was almost as if Gary's memories of Glenn were reserved in a special area of his brain, an area left intact, triggered only when Glenn was around.

That summer, Glenn and Alexis stayed at a campground at the edge of Lake Michigan, a serene and beautiful place where the sun glistens on the water. The backdrop is framed by majestic pine trees that sway in the breeze and wave the sun through to dapple the water — quite a contrast from the bustling college campus where Alexis was a professor.

One morning, about a week into their vacation, Gary Senior went to visit them at the campground. I stayed behind to study for an exam.

I brewed some coffee, sat down at our dining room table, and had barely read five pages when I heard the door slam. It was Gary Senior.

"Something's happened to Glenn!" he exclaimed, gasping between breaths.

"What's wrong?" I asked.

"The ambulance is bringing him to the hospital," he said. "I brought Gary home so I could go see what they have to say."

My eyes widened. "Oh no, what happened?" I asked, following closely behind Gary Senior as he scurried back to the car.

"Glenn collapsed at the campground," he said. "He's conscious, but he looked pale and frightened." Gary Senior hurriedly shoved his way into the car, then rolled down the window. "I'll call you from the hospital when I learn more."

It was strange. Glenn had always seemed very healthy compared to his brother, Gary Senior. I couldn't imagine anything but a sudden accident bringing down this spry man.

At the hospital, doctors discovered a leaking aortic aneurysm. Glenn was in serious condition. He was transported by ambulance to Marquette General Hospital, 65 miles away. Alexis and I followed the ambulance. She was tense and extremely upset. My husband stayed behind with Gary.

Midway to Marquette, we stopped at a country bar to call the hospital for an update. The jukebox box was blaring in the background, and I strained to hear the doctor.

"Glenn's condition is extremely grave," he warned. "Glenn received blood during transport, and we are prepping him for surgery."

I dropped Alexis at the hospital and headed off to my exam. Northern Michigan University was just across the street. I wrote the best exam I could then returned to Alexis at the hospital for our vigil in the surgery waiting room. Alexis' brown eyes reflected fear and turmoil. Her clasped hands cradled her protruding belly as if to protect her unborn child.

We heard from one of the nurses that Glenn survived the surgery. Soon thereafter the doctor came to the waiting room. Presuming I was Glenn's wife, he approached me. I motioned for him to address Alexis, and he began to explain: "Your husband is by no means out of danger. This surgery carries a high mortality rate when the aneurysm has already ruptured. The next 48 hours will be critical."

The surgery was on Thursday; by Saturday afternoon, the doctors were giving a thumbs-up for Glenn's survival. Though his kidneys had not responded, they planned to start dialysis two days later, on Monday.

That evening, my husband traveled to Marquette for a hospital visit. He returned home late. Though exhausted, he seemed relieved that the worst was over.

He was barely home an hour when the hospital called.

"Glenn's condition has taken a negative turn," the nurse said. "Someone should be here with his wife."

I left for the hospital joined by Vicki, who had driven to

our house earlier that day from her home north of Milwaukee. Glenn was her favorite uncle, and they had a close relationship. My husband stayed with Gary, in part because of his own precarious cardiac condition; he knew the excitement could trigger a heart attack or stroke.

At the hospital, we greeted Alexis and then looked in on Glenn. His extremities were swollen to such an extent that his skin looked transparent. He was still awake, but one eye had dilated, indicating possible brain damage.

On Sunday morning, at 6:00 a.m., Glenn slipped into a coma and died. Alexis was by his side, talking to him sweetly and softly about their unborn child, about their dogs, and about heaven. "Jesus wants you, Glenn," she said in a soft, whispery voice. "Go peacefully. I want you too, Glenn, but we must abide by God's plan. I love you."

Vicki and I stood in the doorway listening to Alexis' last words to Glenn. Both of us were blinded by tears.

Later that week, Jeff traveled from Washington, D.C. to attend the private family service for Glenn. On Saturday morning, July 20, 1991, Jeff delivered the following eulogy, holding his 16-month-old daughter Mary Pat who had darted up to the podium after him:

> We have all experienced different slices of Glenn; we each have our unique perspective. To have known him as a brother is perhaps not the same as to have known him as an uncle, a husband, or an in-law; yet there is very much a common denominator to the impressions he left on all of our minds.
>
> We can all agree that Glenn had the gift of a conversationalist — the gift of gab. He could sit down and talk the whole morning about nothing or anything; he could talk sports or politics; he could talk about issues of world importance or those inconsequential with the same amount of enthusiasm and intensity.
>
> He would discuss, listen, argue, dissect, brainstorm, and tell stories; and woven throughout was his unique — at times even outlandish — but always very active and good-natured sense of humor.
>
> When we think of Glenn we think of things nautical —

sailing and the Merchant Marine Academy. We think of pickups, campers, and small English sports cars, particularly the older, less-complicated models that Glenn could take apart and put back together in the same day. We think of his ever-present baseball cap — the wearing of which apparently is a fondness cultivated in only slightly differing degrees by all the male offspring of Vida and Stanton Senior.

We think of his likeness for coffee, cigarettes, and German Shepherd-type watchdogs — and a general likeness for animals. We think of the family historian; knowledge of *exactly* where Thomas Edison fits into our family tree is probably gone with the passing of Glenn.

One hallmark of Glenn's personality was his fondness for, communication with, and ability to inspire kids of all ages. Glenn was really a kid at heart. We think, too, of his sense of frugality; he led a simple and uncomplicated life. Perhaps he knew something about life that most of us don't.

In all, Glenn had a sincere interest in people. As Vicki said, "He is someone you could always count on." And Gary Jr.: "He's a nice guy — a person who would always help you." Both Dave and my mom mentioned his love for kids and dogs. And as my dad, his brother, said this morning: "A person who loves kids and dogs can't be all that bad."

Glenn was down to earth; and now that he is no longer on this earth, may God be kind to his soul.

Glenn's death evoked a normal grieving reaction from Gary. He was deeply moved by the service. With tears in his eyes, Gary said, "I can't believe Glenn is dead!" Perhaps he was overcome by other emotions, but for a good hour or so Gary did not perseverate at all about his age or the year. That was the last — and perhaps the only — time since his brain injury that Gary spent a full waking hour without perseverating.

The next week, Alexis left to go back to her teaching job at Ball State University. She departed with the camper, the two dogs ("Teeper" and "Little One"), and the anticipation of birthing Glenn's child. I admired her strength as I waved good-bye.

Despite everything, and though my time and energy

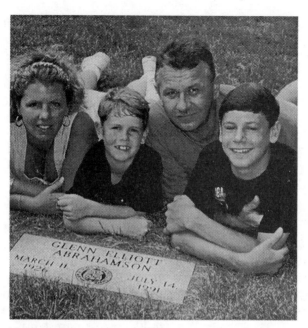

Vicki, Zachary, Dave, and Graham visit Glenn's grave
site, 1992.

seemed limited, I continued my summer classes.

That summer I also requested some of Gary's medical
records, including those from the cardiologist who treated Gary
ten months before his tragedy. After reviewing the records, I
suspected that something wasn't right. That night, I lay in
bed thinking: *I need to contact a lawyer to see if Gary has a
case.*

October 1991 would mark four years since the tragedy
occurred. I knew that every state had a statute of limitations
that limits the time in which a suit can be brought; the purpose is to encourage prompt presentation of claims, presumably while evidence is readily available and witnesses' memories are fresh. So, if Gary *did* have a medical malpractice
case, I knew it ought to be brought sooner than later.

For a couple of days, I wrestled with the idea of a lawsuit.
Contacting a lawyer would probably lead nowhere, I thought.
*Besides, could I afford the diversion from my accelerated sum-
mer classes? No, I'm not going to take the time,* I decided.

That decision was short-lived, however. The next few

nights I woke up nagged by my thoughts: *Gary is incapacitated. He can't do this for himself. A successful lawsuit could be his ticket to badly needed yet very expensive therapy. I've got to be diligent.* Yet, at the time, it really seemed far-fetched.

Nevertheless, I contacted an attorney in Kansas, a man recommended by a local law firm. "Send me all your Michigan medical records and I will collect all the Kansas medical records," he said. "We'll take a look at it and see if the case has merit."

I sent the records off, which if nothing else relieved my thoughts: *Now I've done my duty as an advocate and a mother. It's out of my hands and out of my head. Now I can focus exclusively on classes and Gary's daily care.*

About this time I also began to explore the idea of establishing myself as Gary's legal guardian. His admission into the hospital for heart surgery underscored the possible need to establish one. Back then, the doctor allowed Gary, notwithstanding his cognitive difficulties, to sign the medical consent form. However, I wondered if there would come a time when someone would deem him incapable of signing — either a consent form or a contract — and thereby deny him some service or opportunity that was clearly in his best interest. Also, I reasoned, Gary would need a guardian appointed for the medical malpractice suit, assuming that the case has merit. Besides, there was little reason not to establish a guardianship since Gary Senior and I had by now reconciled ourselves to caring for Gary the rest of our lives — or until there no longer was a need. Finally, a legal guardianship was, at this point, a formality; we were already *de facto* his guardian.

In June, I got the paperwork underway for the guardianship. By August, Gary and I were scheduled for a guardianship hearing before a local judge.

"Gary do you want your mother to be your guardian," the judge asked.

"Yes, I do," Gary responded.

The judge asked Gary several questions that day. Gary rose to the occasion. He behaved appropriately during the entire proceeding — so appropriately, in fact, that I secretly wondered whether the judge would begin to question why he needed a guardian at all!

After the summer semester ended, the Kansas attorney called.

"I'm still looking at the records," he said. "At this point, I need to talk to Gary's wife Kristine to question her about some facts."

"I don't know where she lives," I responded, "nor do I have a phone number; but I will try, through her brother, to get that information for you."

Her brother would not relinquish any information but agreed to contact Kris with the message to call the attorney.

The fall semester started. As part of the social work curriculum at the University, I was required to complete a field internship. I chose the local Community Mental Health Office. They placed me under the supervision of the prevention coordinator, charged with awareness and prevention duties. My tasks were varied and interesting. I attended many interagency meetings and became familiar with local issues.

About this time, I also initiated a weekly column in the local press. In it, I attempted to raise the general level of awareness of such societal problems as depression, drugs, divorce, and suicide. On many occasions, I wrote about traumatic brain injury, its life-long implications, the struggle for services, and legislation to address the problem. I welcomed the opportunity to underscore the importance of not over-relying on expensive institutional care, especially when families — empowered with financial or other assistance from the state — could provide in-home care for victims of brain injury.

In September, Alexis delivered a beautiful baby girl. She named her Elli (Glenn's middle name was Elliott).

By the first part of October 1991, the attorney called: "I have discovered that the statute of limitations can be extended if a person is incapacitated as a result of the malpractice." This was great news for Gary.

Under Kansas law, the statute of limitations requires a medical malpractice claim to be brought within two years of the doctor's harmful act (in Gary's case the harmful act occurred on December 2, 1986, when the doctor wrongfully diagnosed his condition). But, if the injury is not reasonably

ascertainable until sometime after the doctor's harmful act —
and Gary's injury was not ascertained until his heart stoppage on October 25, 1987 — then the claim must be brought
within two years of discovering the injury (by October 25, 1989)
but no longer than four years after the doctor's harmful act
(by December 2, 1990).

In short, the ordinary statute of limitations had run out.
But there was an exception under Kansas law. This exception
extended the statute of limitations for persons incapacitated
due to the medical negligence to eight years after the doctor's
harmful act (or until December 2, 1994) or one year after the
person's incapacitation is cured or removed. In Gary's case,
his incapacitation likely would be considered removed once I
was appointed his guardian in August 1991. So, all of this
meant that we had until August 1992 to file a claim.

Ironically, had Gary lost both eyes and all four limbs due
to medical negligence, his injuries probably would have been
time barred by October 1991, when I first contacted the lawyer. It was the nature of his injury — an incapacitating brain
injury — which saved his suit from the statute of limitations.
We almost learned the hard way that if you are harmed by
someone and the law permits you to recover damages, don't
wait too long before hiring an attorney to bring your claim.

About that time, Gary received a letter from Kris. She
and the boys were planning a trip to Escanaba near the end of
October. Gary and Kris' wedding anniversary — October 28 —
was approaching, and she indicated that they would go out to
dinner.

But Kris didn't visit Gary that October. Instead, on November 5, she filed for divorce.

I was at school when the notice came. My husband was
puzzled when he saw the sheriff's deputy approaching the
house.

"Is Patt Abrahamson here?" the sheriff's deputy asked.

"No, she's at school," my husband replied.

"Would you have her come down to the sheriff's office and
pick up a summons?" the deputy said courteously. "Or call
and we will come over with it one more time."

Later that day, I picked up the legal papers. In some

respects, it was just a formality. Their marriage had ended long before this.

There wasn't any point in discussing it with Gary. I tried to shield him from even temporary grief.

Another Christmas neared. Vicki and her family drove to Escanaba from their home north of Milwaukee to spend the holidays with us. Jeff spent Christmas day with his family in Virginia, but then flew to Escanaba with his daughter Mary Pat to join us for several days.

We doted on Mary Pat and marveled at how smart our granddaughter was. We reacted, I believe, like most grandparents. Though Gary couldn't help his behavior — including his perseverative questions about his age and the year — it was all foreign to Mary Pat. Though not yet two-years old, she knew Gary's behavior was unusual and tended to shy away from him. Even if she was laughing or smiling the moment before Gary came into the room, her behavior changed with his presence. She would strike a frown, subtly move away from Gary, or seek the comfort of another person.

Gary recognized her attempt to avoid him, which tended to increase his agitation. Like a German Shepherd that can sense when someone is scared, Gary would then focus greater attention on her. He'd say, "Why won't she answer me?" or "Why does she have that look on her face?"

Mary Pat would run to her father and sit in his lap. She was especially frightened if Gary raised his voice. We were all cognizant of the problem, and made a concerted effort to separate the two "kids."

Spring 1992 marked three years since Gary came to live with us. It had been three years of investigation, experimentation, and frustration — tempered only by hope, love, and prayer. Gradually, the situation began to stabilize. The burden was more bearable due to a confluence of causes. Among them, respite care was key; it provided for more planned and structured activities, which translated into less agitation at home; it improved the quality of our interaction with Gary.

We were learning — primarily through trial and error — what to say, and when, and what to ignore. We discovered how best to access information without intimidating him. We also learned not to take things personally and not to respond with hurt feelings. Gary Senior and I had every incentive to search for techniques to decrease Gary's frustration, thereby improving the quality of our lives. And we seized upon every such opportunity.

Things weren't yet serene; peace was not yet at hand. But, a cease-fire had definitely come about. We were able to withdraw from the combat zone, enter the demilitarized zone, and rest up for possible future skirmishes.

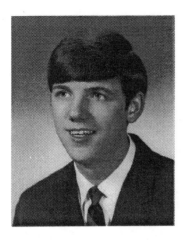

Gary's high school graduation picture, 1968.

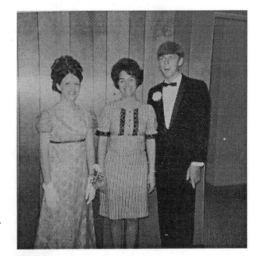

Vicki, Patt, and Gary, 1968.

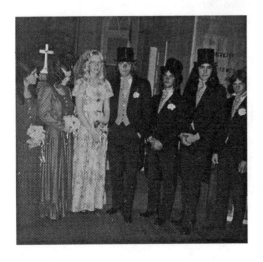

Gary's wedding. Vicki (far left), Gary and Kris (middle), Jeff (far right), 1972.

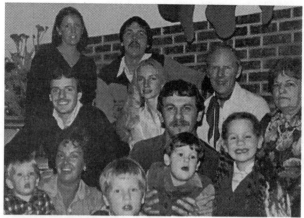

Christmas 1980. Vicki and Gary (top row). Jeff, Kris, Dave, Gary Senior, Grandma Flath (middle row). Leif, Patt, Arlo, Graham, Heather (bottom row).

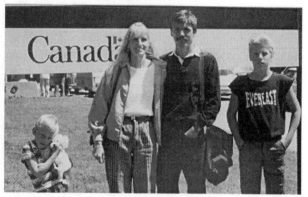

Gary, Kris, Arlo, Leif, and Chantilly Lace on vacation. Sault Ste. Marie, Ontario, 1985.

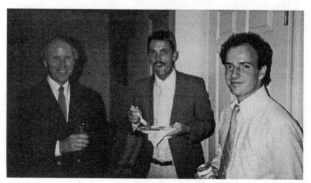

Gary Senior, Gary, and Jeff, 1985.

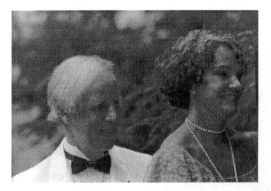

Gary Senior and Patt, 1985.

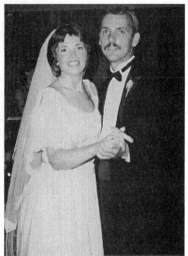

Gary and Jeff's new bride Peggy, 1985.

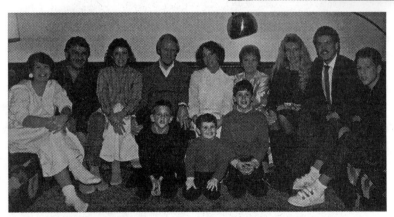

Christmas 1986. Seated from left to right: Heather, Dave, Vicki, Gary
Senior, Patt, Grandma Flath, Kris, Gary, Arlo. Kneeling from left to right:
Leif, Zachary, Graham.

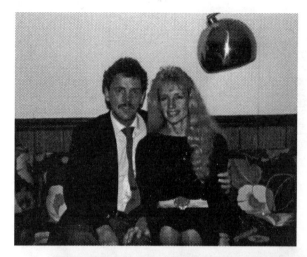

Gary and Kris,
Christmas 1986.

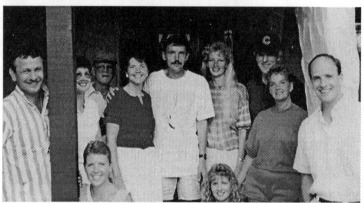

Summer 1988. Standing left to right: Dave, Alexis, Glenn, Peggy,
Gary, Kris, Gary Senior, Patt, Jeff. Kneeling left to right: Vicki,
Heather.

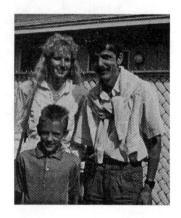

Gary, Kris, Leif, 1988.

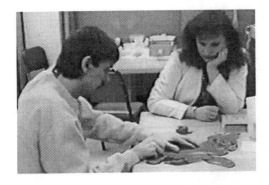

Gary with occupational therapist, 1988.

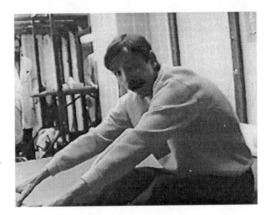

Gary in physical therapy, 1988.

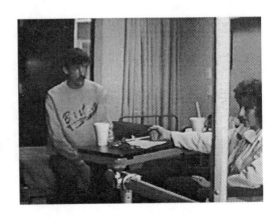

Gary with speech pathologist, 1988.

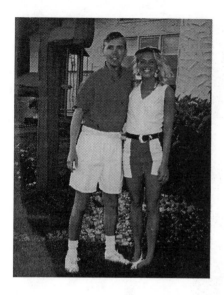

Gary with Carmella, his aide and friend, 1993.

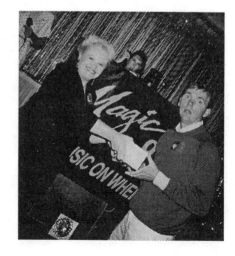

Gary receives door prize at his 25-year high school class reunion, 1993.

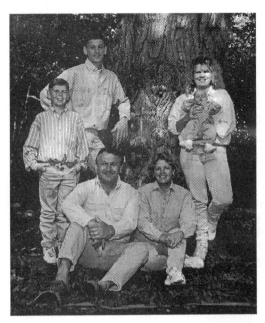

Vicki's family, 1994. Dave and Vicki (sitting); Zachary, Graham, Heather and her baby Gabrielle.

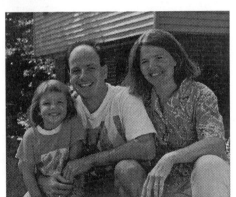

Jeff, Peggy, and Mary Pat, 1994.

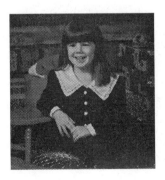

Glenn and Alexis' daughter Elli, 1995.

BRAIN INJURY: A FAMILY TRAGEDY

12

BUREAUCRATIC
BULLFEATHERS

If men be good, government cannot be bad.
- William Penn

Before the traumatic incident, we knew nothing about brain injury; we had little experience dealing with the social services system; we knew next to nothing about government delivery of benefits for those in our society with special needs.

We soon learned that seeking public services for a person with a brain injury is more than a challenge; for us, it was a baptism-under-fire introduction to the social services bureaucracy — sort of like learning how to walk during a foot race.

There exists a plethora of agencies, each with its own expertise and methods. As to common societal needs, we have developed well-known methods to access government services. For example, if you: have an emergency medical problem, go to the hospital; see a fire, call the fire department; witness a crime, call the police; are recently laid off, apply for unemployment and possibly retraining programs; are elderly, receive social security and medicare; are poor, apply for food stamps and Medicaid; are poor with children, apply for aid to families with dependent children (AFDC); are a veteran, use the services of the Veterans Administration; are caring for someone that is either mentally ill or developmentally disabled, use the services of the local Community Mental Health office.

But, where do you go for your family member with a brain injury? There is no Department of Brain Injury, no program specifically set up to provide aid to families with dependent brain injured individuals. It was, at first, difficult just to determine which agency I should be calling.

After a while, it seemed as if they were cutting my son up into different pieces: see Community Mental Health for his mental and social needs; see Michigan Rehabilitation Services for rehabilitation needs; see Social Security for funds for basic needs; see doctors for his medical needs.

As I ran from one agency to another, I often wondered, *Why do I have to give the same information to all these agencies? Couldn't they coordinate somehow so that families overburdened with primary care don't have fill out multiple forms asking for the same information?* Seeing how the system worked — or didn't work — for Gary made me want to advocate at the local, state, and national levels for the needs of *all* brain injury survivors.

While Gary was still in the hospital — before he came to live with us — I got my first experience in dealing with *the system.* Because Gary's private medical insurance would eventually run out, the social worker at Marquette General Hospital advised me to apply for Medicaid.

Medicaid, a means-tested program to provide medical services to low-income individuals, is a joint federal-state program. States, on average, pay less than half of the costs to administer the program and are able, as long as they stay within broad federal parameters, to set benefit and eligibility levels.

I went to the Department of Social Services in Escanaba where the staff asked me to fill out an application form that resembled a small book, then return it when complete. Now, I consider myself a person of at least average intelligence; yet, I was unable to complete the forms. The agency apparently was aware of this potential hurdle to accessing services because the bottom of the application stated clearly and in bold print: "If you are unable to complete this application, the law states that the agency must help you."

So, I asked for help. I was greeted with very eloquent non-verbal messages from agency personnel; they seemed irritated and exasperated that *anyone* would need help with this form! Experiencing their ire was, apparently, the undeclared price of receiving help from them.

After the application was complete and submitted, agency staff reviewed it. It didn't take long before I was curtly told that Gary did not meet the program requirements. At that, I insisted on seeing the department head. He looked at the application, then looked up.

"This accident happened in Kansas," he said. "Why is he here?"

"Well, Gary and his wife were raised in Escanaba — both graduated from high school here," I responded. "Gary's family is going to move back to Michigan."

"He should go back to Kansas," he blurted. "This is their responsibility!"

I told the social worker at Marquette General what happened. Appalled, she set up an appointment with the Department of Social Services office in Marquette. There, I am happy to say, I was treated with dignity. In fact, the intake worker had a son who also had a brain injury. *She*, no doubt, understood our situation, and we were thankful for that.

Through the Marquette office, Gary was deemed to have met the income requirements and *did* qualify for Michigan Medicaid. However, Michigan Medicaid reimburses the hospital at a lower rate than full-pay private insurance does for the same services. About the time Gary's private insurance ended, Marquette General discharged him because he was "not making progress." That may have been just a coincidence; even so, I couldn't help but wonder whether the lower reimbursement rate had — at least on the margin — anything to do with his discharge.

My next encounter with the local Department of Social Services was equally as awkward, just as unpleasant. Providing for Gary's 24-hour daily care limited our income possibilities. So, I applied under another program for some home help to assist us financially and otherwise. This time, a local supervisor said, "Don't think that we're going to provide babysitting services for your son." This was the same agency that told us Gary should move back to Kansas. For a split second, I felt what it must have been like to live under the old Soviet regime, dependent upon despotic bureaucrats for housing and other necessities. Thank God these ignoble agents of our government normally have but limited influence on our lives. If it were otherwise, rebellion and revolution — I assure you — would be just around the corner!

They seemed unenlightened about the needs of people with brain injuries and appeared wholly unconcerned about our plight. I wondered if their self-appointed function was to look askance at people with legitimate needs. Apparently they had their own list of legitimate public needs and caring for a person with a brain injury at home wasn't yet on that list. Perhaps they were more concerned about conserving budget dollars than providing public services. If so, they apparently failed to consider that the cost to the State to institutionalize Gary would, no doubt, be far greater than whatever assistance we were requesting to care for him in our home.

I complained to a staffer in the headquarters office in Lansing who was quite sympathetic. She was familiar with one of the bureaucrats, whose reputation apparently preceded him. "I understand," she said. "We have received numerous complaints about that individual, but there's not much we can do but wait for him to retire." What a sad commentary on our bureaucratic system.

In fairness to him, however, he was probably allocating State resources under general statutes, regulations, and guidelines which were written to address — not brain injury — but more common societal needs. At worst, brain injury simply fell between programmatic cracks. At best, we had to rely on bureaucrats to use humane discretion to both understand the needs of brain injury victims and their families and then find an appropriate program or regulation to allow that need to be met. Perhaps that is too much to expect. A better approach would be for legislators to recognize these needs and write them into law.

Unless state or federal statutes or regulations explicitly provide for the provision of services to victims of brain injury and their families, one is forced to pay homage to the altar of bureaucratic discretion. Bestowed with vast amounts of autonomy, bureaucrats act as gatekeepers, wielding significant power over the lives of those in need of government services.

That is not to say that bestowing them with appropriate amounts of discretion is bad. In the proper hands, discretion can spawn efficient and creative solutions to problems. In fact, there are many capable, responsive, skillful, and dedicated public servants that work public miracles on a daily basis.

But, the unresponsive or unprofessional bureaucrat can be frustrating indeed. Perhaps you caught the bureaucrat on a bad day; or perhaps he or she resents you because you're informed, competent, and assertive; or perhaps he or she loses patience with you because you're, at least initially, uninformed. Any one of these circumstances can be fatal to getting services.

Agency counselors have been known to pass the buck with a comment like: "My supervisor would never approve this request," even though the counselor has the authority to act without such supervisory approval. Most of us, unwise to the system, simply accept such statements as fact, thus wiping out any due process power we may have had.

Then, too, there is the Biblical adage: "Ask, and you shall receive." We may be eligible for all kinds of services — ramps, personal care assistants, wheelchairs, occupational therapy assessments, college tuition, etc. — but if we do not ask for a *specific* service, there is no guarantee the counselor will inform us that it is available.

While fiscal responsibility may legitimately drive *some* of this behavior, it is too often the case that prejudices, personalities, and other unprofessional considerations enter into bureaucratic judgments.

There is another factor that works against accessing services for the brain injury community. Many people, including those in charge of rationing public services, simply don't understand the cognitive, social, or psychological implications of brain injury. After all, people with a brain injury don't always look needy. They may not have crutches or need a wheelchair. They may have all of their limbs. They may not walk with a cane or be guided by a seeing-eye dog. Since we live in a small community where Gary is seen about town regularly, it wouldn't surprise me if agency personnel developed an impression — simply based on their own visual examination — that Gary was not particularly deserving of public assistance.

If so, then it's no wonder that bureaucratic discretion was exercised as it was — not in Gary's favor.

Recognizing these and other potential hurdles to accessing public assistance for people with a brain injury, I decided to simply bypass the agencies and enlist the help of our then-U.S. Congressman Bob Davis. Congressman Davis contacted then-Michigan Department of Social Services Director C. Patrick Babcock about our case, which led to Gary's evaluation at Mary Free Bed to determine whether he was an appropriate candidate for a transitional living program for traumatic brain injury (TBI) survivors. Gary didn't make the program, but the series of contacts apparently may have paid off locally; it wasn't until *after* this series of contacts that the local Department of Social Services approved my request for home help. For me, this served to underscore a time-honored cliche — the squeaky wheel *does* get the grease.

Receiving this and other publicly-funded relief tremendously lessened our burden. Had this type of assistance come earlier, it may have helped keep Gary's family together. We'll never know. I do know one thing, however; because of the dearth of programs for brain injury clients, we had to navigate the system, uncover potential programs that could help, then tenaciously fight to allow Gary to access them.

The whole process raised my consciousness about the unmet needs of other people in my position — especially those less skilled or persistent than I. In any case, the lessons I learned help to kindle my interest in educating, advocating, and helping to produce systemic change for victims of brain injury and their families.

There are a lot of agencies out there — some help with income stabilization, others with assistive devices, or home adaptations, or job retraining, or mental health. If you have an unmet need, it's a good idea to keep searching until you find an agency that deals with that, and then keep on asking until you get services.

But, there is generally no coordinated effort to meet the needs of individuals with a brain injury. So, even if you do run into a bureaucrat that is friendly, wants to help, it is not the end of the puzzle. That's because searching for the right programs for an individual with a brain injury is sometimes akin to shopping in the kind of big, ugly warehouse-type store they used to have in the deep South: Uncle Bo-Diddly's General Discount Store, with shovels and bicycles hanging from the ceiling over party supplies, furniture, and diapers, all jumbled together with nails, perfume, and whatever else the store owner could get wholesale, the kind of place where the clerk is likely to say, "Yeah, I think we have some of that stuff over here. Or was it over there? Or was that last week? I don't know. Why don't you look around? We've got a lot of good stuff here. Can you use one of our handy-dandy widgets?"

A caseworker from the Department of Social Services visited me quarterly. Though he was a very nice gentlemen, he too was clearly unfamiliar with TBI. One of the roles that a caseworker plays is to help victims access services — not only from his agency but other agencies as well.

Unfortunately, he didn't know what services were available or even what services were needed. Though he had a four-year degree, it was not in the human services area. I joked with him that *I* should be getting a salary for case management because, in effect, I *was* Gary's case manager; I was the one seeking out available services, dealing with different agencies for his cognitive, medical and financial needs.

In early 1992, the Department of Social Services informed me that the agency was implementing new guidelines for the home care program. One of the reasons that Gary requires 24-hour daily care is that he needs to be cued, or coached, to perform certain basic functions, such as showering and shaving. While he can physically perform these activities himself, he needs to be reminded to do them, then coached to completion. The new functional assessment guidelines, as they were called, were going to eliminate cuing from the home care program. That, in turn, meant our financial assistance for home care would be pruned. Yet, cuing is critical to Gary's performance of everyday duties.

Nevertheless, Gary was scheduled for a functional needs assessment under the new program requirements. The agency's case manager met with me to ascertain Gary's level of functionality. We sat at the dining room table in our family home. Reading from a questionnaire drawn up by the Department, he began.

"Can Gary lift his fork to his mouth?"

"Yes," I replied, "but *you* and I both know that he would begin to lose weight if he were not cued to eat."

"I understand, but we are only looking at function here," he replied.

"Can he toilet himself?" he continued.

"Yes, but he needs help to clean himself after a bowel movement," I answered, feeling a sense of panic rise in my throat.

"I understand, but we are only interested in function," he explained. "*Can he do it?*"

"Yes." My panic was slowly turning to despair.

"Can Gary shower himself?"

By now, the whole exercise seemed so silly, so pointless.

"Yes, but he wouldn't do it unless he is cued," I said, feeling myself beginning to get angry.

"I understand, but we are only interested in whether he can physically shower himself."

Finally, I cut to the chase:

"*Yes,*" I said. "Physically, Gary *can* do almost everything — but his cognitive impairment would hinder his initiating even getting out of bed in the morning."

The bureaucrat agreed, but again reiterated, "The new functional assessment guidelines only evaluate function."

He subsequently concluded that based on the new guidelines, Gary's home help would be drastically cut.

Gary was up for a review in December 1992, but the case manager's supervisor insisted that the review be moved up to August instead. I filed a protest.

In the meantime, I contacted the Brain Injury Association of Michigan. At their prompting, I contacted the Protection and Advocacy Service, a publicly-funded group that helps people advocate their case before State agencies. They informed me that many others had contacted them once the State began to implement their new guidelines to achieve cost containment. Most had filed protests. In response, the Protection and Advocacy Service contacted heads of the appropriate departments.

For my part, I wrote a letter to the Directors of the Department of Mental Health and the Department of Social Services. That letter read, in part, as follows:

> We are trying desperately to prevent institutionalization of our son Gary (41), who is brain injured.
>
> He needs twenty-four hour care due to memory problems and a number of other functional deficits, including cognition impairment, executive function deficits, and a serious perseveration problem.
>
> Originally, I was refused any home help assistance from the local Department of Social Services. It was only after Congressman Bob Davis contacted the Director of the Department of Social Services that help was forthcoming.
>
> Based on the new functional needs assessment guidelines, Gary's home care help is scheduled to be drastically cut. Providing assistance for cuing saves the State monies by preventing institutionalization. Evidence has shown that the system promotes expensive residential care to the exclusion of more appropriate and affordable in-home care.
>
> I have written to Congressmen Bob Davis, Carl Pursell, and John Dingell asking them to co-sponsor federal legislation that would increase brain injury awareness and assistance. To further create awareness, I also write a local column on social issues, frequently addressing brain injury.
>
> So far, I have managed to channel my anger in a positive way — to address systemic changes. In my opinion, the Michigan Mental Health Code needs to define brain injury as a distinct population. Many states simply include brain injury under developmental disabilities. Although Michigan's Mental Health Code addresses "organic brain and other neurological impairments," it gives priority to the mentally-impaired and developmentally-disabled populations. Locally, I have been told a hundred times: "Too bad, but Gary falls through the cracks."
>
> If the system is truly interested in cost containment, it would promote programs that help keep people like Gary in the home.

The Michigan Department of Social Services Director responded:

> Thank you for your letter of March 10, 1992. I want to compliment you for the work you are performing on behalf of your son, Gary. His care requirements are tremendous and your efforts to meet his needs are exemplary.
>
> As you know, the Governor is struggling with severe budget deficits and this undoubtedly will impact on our Department's program operations at some point in the future.
>
> In the meantime, I am pleased that our Adult Home Help Services Program has [been able to assist Gary].

The Michigan Department of Mental Health Director responded:

> I have reviewed the letter and attached material sent in your March 10, 1992 letter. The difficulty you have found in trying to get support for your son brings home to me the lack of clarity of roles and responsibilities the Department of Mental Health has with closed head injuries and the subsequent rehabilitative needs. I will be raising your concerns as well as similar cases with Gerald Miller, Director of the Department of Social Services. We have agreed that there are many overlapping services and needs between our two Departments that need to be better coordinated. I believe that this is one of those high need areas and will give it a top priority to find better ways of dealing with these issues in the future. ...

Ultimately, implementation of the new functional guidelines were dropped — at least in our case as well as in similar ones. Perhaps a rash of protests, coupled with intervention by Protection and Advocacy Services, prompted the State to re-evaluate its position. I'm not sure. In any case, our home help was continued.

Later that same year, I had the dubious distinction of once again coming face to face with *the system.* I learned that speech therapy was now available through the local Community Mental Health Office. The PASS program, which had made it possible to hire someone to engage Gary in recreation therapy and community re-entry activities, had already reduced our day-to-day stress levels; now we wanted to see Gary get the speech and occupational therapy he clearly needed. So, I re-applied to the Community Mental Heath agency for these services on Gary's behalf. In order to officially determine Gary's needs, the agency arranged for him to meet with a psychiatrist. The psychiatrist had this to say, in part:

Gary was alert. He paid attention to me. I talked to him alone for a period of time. He became somewhat upset and agitated. He was lost, wasn't sure where he was. He was concerned and confused. His hands were icy cold. He started to get louder and louder. I had his parents come in and join us. He continued to get somewhat louder with them. He was [perseverating about] his age ... At one point he did say that he was sad and I tried to get [him to elaborate, but he would] go right back to his age. Before I asked him about the sadness, which he came up with fairly voluntarily, we had been conversing fairly comfortably; when I tried to make an attempt to pursue the sadness, it seemed to be fairly obvious that he would just [want to talk about] age ... [it was unclear] whether he wouldn't let me or whether he was unable to access that material. ...

This is an individual who has suffered a massive brain insult and who has continued to show some very slow, but progressive recovery. He is being monitored very closely by his [parents, who] have really created an environment that is very appropriate for Gary and help him in every way they can. They desperately want some services for this gentleman to try to help maximize his abilities and potential. In questioning him today, I was surprised at the voluntary statement from him that he was sad and was amazed at how any attempt to pursue that resulted in perseveration on age, which almost seemed intentional to prevent me from getting any more information ... He certainly does have some difficulties with speech [and] some problems with memory. Services such as occupational therapy and speech therapy, I think, would be appropriate for him; it is a possibility that there may be some depression present that he is not talking about. I don't [think] the use of medication is appropriate at the present time.

After the evaluation, I waited weeks for a response. None

came. Finally, I made an appointment with a Community Mental Health Departmental Supervisor. I got right to the point.

"When will the psychiatrist-recommended therapies for Gary begin," I asked.

"Your case is going before the Board this evening," he responded. "Your son's case falls between the cracks. By definition, he's not developmentally disabled nor is he mentally ill. Funding is scarce, and according to the Michigan Mental Health Code, brain injury is not a priority."

After that, I re-read appropriate sections of the Michigan Mental Health Code. In 1992, the statutory language required a county mental health program to address at least one of five areas — mental illness, developmental disability, brain injury, alcoholism, or substance abuse. But, the Code said, "priority shall be given to the areas of mental illness and developmental disabilities." Gary would have qualifed as developmentally disabled — and thereby been afforded priority status — if his mental impairment had, according to the Code, manifested itself before he turned 22 years old. In the end, the staff recommended against providing services to Gary.

The whole thing saddened me profoundly. Another refusal of services. Another dead end. Then, my sorrow turned to anger. *I will attend that meeting*, I thought. *I will personally bring my son's plight before the Board: my son, who can't advocate for himself; my son, who falls through the cracks; my son, who is not considered a priority.*

The meeting was scheduled for early that evening. At home, we had a quicker than usual dinner and made arrangements for someone to stay with Gary. With little time to spare, we headed off to the meeting location on the outskirts of town. As we drove across town, I began to reflect on the situation.

Gazing out the window, I noticed a family walking their dog in the pleasant but brisk spring evening. They seemed so breezy and carefree — so happy and animated. By contrast, I felt troubled, annoyed, and perplexed.

I was troubled by the colossal effort required to access appropriate services for individuals with a brain injury. I was annoyed to think that I probably would not have been informed about the impending Board meeting but for my persistence.

And I was perplexed by humanity; in so many ways we are altruistic, charitable, and compassionate. Through public programs and private associations, we fund the rehabilitation of drug abusers; we help habitual criminals gain college degrees; we spend money to protect birds and other wildlife; we spend countless hours and dollars on things like restoring old buildings. Yet my son, a human being with needs, "falls through the cracks" and "is not a priority."

At the meeting site, we parked the car. Lugging my purse and a stack of papers in one hand, I clutched my husband's arm with other, and we walked toward the attractive, modern structure that housed the social services and community mental health offices. Once inside, we made our way down one long hallway, then another, pausing only for a moment to greet a just-arriving Board member.

We entered the Board room where most of the eight or so Board members were already seated in plush chairs behind a nicely appointed semi-circular table on a raised platform. Two staff members sat at a small, modest rectangular table to the side. As the meeting was about to start, Gary Senior and I were the only members of the public present.

Soon the meeting was brought to order. The Board disposed of several items unrelated to our plight. Then came our issue. The administrator of the Delta County Mental Heath Program began by advising the other Board members that there had been "some service requests" for persons with a brain injury in the county; though we were sitting in the front row, he chose to keep it impersonal, not recognize us or link us to the request. He explained that staff had denied these requests due to a combination of budget problems and the State Code. Toward the end of the meeting, I asked to make a statement.

"My son Gary has a brain injury," I began. "I requested speech therapy for him, which would cost approximately $6,000 for one year. I certainly understand why your agency elects to provide services to substance abusers even though they — like victims of brain injury — aren't considered *a priority* under the Michigan Mental Health Code either; but I have trouble understanding why similar services are denied to my son, who is not a substance abuser but is a member of this community who has a brain injury and needs help."

A few Board members were sympathetic. One spoke up: "Why can't we apply for a Program Revision Request (PRR) and see if we can get this woman some help?"

Letting that comment hang in the air for a few seconds, the administrator appeared reluctant but then uttered, "Good idea. We could do that." A motion was made and the proposal was adopted. Now it was up to staff to draft the Program Revision Request, then bring it back to the Board for approval.

By the following month, the proposed PRR was completed and placed on the agenda for consideration. I attended the meeting, and obtained a copy of the Program Revision Request, which read, in part:

> In order to meet a community need for the treatment of persons with neurological conditions, we are proposing a PRR that would treat up to 10 residents of Delta County. As you know, people with Alzheimer's Disease and Traumatic Brain Injury and other neurological conditions are not currently treatment priorities in our system. However, these people do exist in our county, often with significant needs for habilitation, case management and possible residential placement.
>
> We are proposing to treat 10 individuals, much like the Developmental Disability Waiver program, by bringing in professional and paraprofessional staff into their current homes in order to habilitate and prevent expensive residential placements. We may also be able to return residents to their homes from current residential programs or nursing homes with this program. In addition to in-home services, there are also case management, day program, respite, and family support components provided for in this proposal. We estimate the total cost for the treatment of these 10 individuals would be $412,700, of which $315,060 would be funded by the State.
>
> The Board understands that neurological impairments are not a priority for service within the Mental Health Code. However, the Board also believes that the principles of community-based care and "least restrictive" alternative are as applicable to this potential client group as to persons with mental illness or developmental disabilities. By the services envisioned, we hope to (a) reduce the risk of out-of-home placement and/or (b) assure that the rehabilita-

tive potential of each person is first assessed and then maximized through an appropriate plan of service.

Just like that, with the stroke of a pen, my entreaty for a modest $6,000 suddenly exploded into a major program request totalling $412,700! Given the budgetary climate, such a sum seemed sure to be rejected by the State. Losing patience, I asked agency personnel, "Who put this program request together?" Everyone looked stunned, glancing from one to the other to see who would take credit for the ludicrous proposal destined for denial. No one did.

Frustrated, I then became hyper-critical of the choice of terms used in the PRR. I criticized the use of "habilitate," which means to train someone to acquire a skill for the first time. That term is normally used in the context of the developmentally disabled. "Rehabilitate," which means restoring a person to his or her previous state, is a more appropriate description for treating people with a brain injury. Though I didn't mention it, I was also surprised that they lumped in Alzheimer's victims, who — because of the degenerative nature of their disease — cannot generally be habilitated or rehabilitated.

In any case, the questionable request was forwarded to the State. Months passed. No word. I filed a complaint with the agency's recipients rights worker whose job consists of, among other things, assisting potential recipients to access services through appeals if necessary. She told me that the PRR had been denied several weeks earlier. Again, but for my own persistence, the agency apparently was not planning to inform me of that decision.

Another agency encouraged me to appeal the decision further. By this time, however, I was so discouraged, I dropped it. I was still in school. I was still fully responsible for my son's care, needs, and welfare.

I was beginning to conclude that trying to get services for a loved one with a brain injury in a system devised with other priorities in mind was like trying to fit a square peg in a round hole. You were sure to encounter time, trouble and turmoil; for that, you would be met with resistance, repudiation and rejection. And in the end, you may be left with little more than a bunch of paperwork.

Though on the surface I may have been calmly moving forward like a duck on the water, underneath my legs were working furiously; yet my paddling had only limited effect. My duties were enormous and diverse, and my energy and tenacity had begun to wane. They — the agency, the regulatory process, the statutory language, the *system* — were wearing me down.

13

CHASING ANSWERS

We are not interested in the possibilities of defeat.
- Queen Victoria

Our search for answers through programs, institutions and agencies seemed to be bear only a little fruit. There was more, I was sure, that we could do right at home to help rehabilitate Gary.

I continued to learn all I could about brain injury. At the University library, I found a recently published book that piqued my interest: *Introduction to Cognitive Rehabilitation* by McKay Moore Sohlberg and Catherine A. Mateer. After reading the book, I decided to contact Dr. Sohlberg. She informed me that she would be conducting a workshop later that month at Meriter Hospital in Madison, Wisconsin — just a five-hour drive from our home. Immediately, I shifted into high gear, arranging for Gary's care, registering for the conference, and securing accommodations. The workshop's focus was theory and management techniques for attention deficits, memory impairments, and executive functions. How timely! These were the biggest problem areas for Gary.

Though the workshop was geared toward the medical, research, and rehabilitative professional, attending the conference in the capacity of Gary's primary caretaker proved to be a helpful learning experience.

I already knew that Gary had frontal lobe damage: that such damage almost always occurs after oxygen deprivation. At the workshop, I learned that the frontal lobes, located just behind the forehead, are the most recently developed part of the brain in an evolutionary sense, are the last part of the brain to develop in a maturing individual, and are necessary to organize and regulate behavior necessary to accomplishment. The frontal lobes are critical to the so-called "executive functions" of initiation, planning, organization, self-monitoring, and completion of purposeful activities. As such, frontal lobe damage impairs a person's ability to engage in goal-directed behavior.

This meant that Gary's problem wasn't just a memory problem — it was more insidious, more far-reaching. Moreover, I learned that impairment of these abilities may be present *despite* intact and strong intellectual skills.

It started to make sense. It helped explain Gary's seemingly paradoxical abilities. Gary is fabulous at math problems; he can play chess; he passed a driver's exam; he even corrects his dad's spelling mistakes. Yet, he is unable to complete shaving his face without prompting! Gary had intelligence, but needed assistance to exercise it. Gary didn't lack motivation, even though I had seen one inexperienced therapist act as if that were the case.

I also learned that a person with frontal lobe damage will have difficulty making mental or behavioral shifts. They may verbalize a resolution to a problem but are unable to effect a plan; they are long on solutions, short on execution. Instead, they may perseverate on a single idea or a single action.

I left that workshop eager to search for funding to take Gary to the Good Samaritan Hospital in Puyallup, Washington, where Dr. Sohlberg and Catherine Mateer practiced. Both of these professionals are highly esteemed for their theory and implementation of management techniques to rehabilitate individuals with a brain injury; they seemed to be especially knowledgeable about oxygen-deprivation-induced brain injuries and special rehabilitative techniques for the victims of such injuries.

Once again, I met with Michigan Rehabilitation Services Supervisor John Porter, who had been most helpful in the past. I suggested the following scenario: I could go to Puyallup for two months, learn the techniques, then hire and train aides locally to continue the program at minimum wage. John Porter told me to make the arrangements — that Michigan Rehabilitation Services would help fund the undertaking.

Soon thereafter, I learned that Good Samaritan was not a teaching hospital — they did not have a program to teach the families of victims their techniques for rehabilitation. That quashed my plan to spend two months learning from them. The only option was to admit Gary into the program. However, two or three months would not be adequate they said; Gary would have to go for an extended amount of time — six to twelve months minimum.

Meanwhile, I was also corresponding with Dr. Sohlberg. I described Gary's situation in detail and provided her with clinical reports. She suggested that it would be best if Gary was able to receive training close to home. In one of her letters, she explains:

> ... Gary sounds like he would best benefit from training that is carried out in the same context that the activity will be performed. Given the nature of his brain injury, I would predict that he would have a difficult time generalizing information learned in one context to another setting ...
>
> Ultimately, I think it would be critical to have structured training carried out in Gary's home with you (or whoever would be providing supportive care) to facilitate functioning with the minimum level of cuing. We find family training to be critical to the success of our rehabilitation programs.
>
> I am very impressed that he spends five hours a day out in the community — that is to your and Gary's credit. So many persons in his situation are completely isolated from community activities. I admire your commitment and dedication to maximize Gary's quality of life. My only caution, and I am sure you have heard this before, is that your best support of Gary is to take care of yourself and make sure your own individual needs are being met. A huge congratulations on your pending degree.

I couldn't help but lament the poverty of specialists and clinicians knowledgeable about brain injury in Michigan's Upper Peninsula.

At that point, I met with John Porter from Michigan Rehabilitation Services again.

"John, I am grateful to your agency," I said. "It's the only one that has offered any resources in my efforts to rehabilitate Gary. Where do I go now? Any ideas? Locally, we just don't have any clinicians who are experienced with brain injury."

"I understand Marquette General has revamped their TBI program," John explained.

"What about funding?" I asked.

"Michigan Rehabilitation Services will fund evaluations for Gary," he responded.

I agreed to investigate their new outpatient program, even though Marquette is 65 miles from our home. If necessary, I would make the 130-mile round trip three days a week for Gary's therapy.

As a first step, they wanted to formally evaluate Gary. We took Gary to Marquette for a battery of evaluations. The neuropsychological report indicated that — despite Gary's brain injury — he still scored within the normal intelligence range. He correctly answered a number of general information questions and performed several math calculations, including those that required three-step operations.

However, his attention and concentration skills were found to be seriously impaired as were his memory and learning capabilities. With regard to executive function — the higher organizational, planning, and directing aspects of brain performance — the neuropsychologist noted that his inability to inhibit perseverative questions, such as constantly asking the year and his age, were symptomatic of dysfunctional executive abilities. There was something compelling about these questions, something telling his brain to keep asking them. The neuropsychologist likened his perseverative questioning to a formidable "feedback loop," one which is nearly impossible for him to disrupt, thus making meaningful interactions with others difficult. She identified this internal feedback process as one of Gary's main obstacles to effective utilization of other aspects of cognition. Moreover, she seemed to think that certain remediation strategies could be employed to help him disrupt this internal feedback process.

Gary was also evaluated by speech, physical, and occupational therapists. Though his perseveration was listed as a barrier to treatment, Marquette General's traumatic brain injury program decided to accept Gary in an outpatient program with one caveat — that he would have to be medicated to help control his agitation and perseverative behavior. Since only a doctor or psychiatrist can prescribe medication, Gary was scheduled for a psychiatric evaluation. Excerpts from that evaluation follow:

.... He was treated at one point with some Haldol to try to control some of his more aggressive behaviors. The parents felt that he was overly sedated on Haldol and he was taking, by old records, it appears, .5 to 1 mg. At the same time he was also taking Inderal and Tegretol. ... Mr. Abrahamson is currently living with his parents who have done a good job of extending themselves to take care of him, but who are both older and tiring some in the long siege they have gone through in helping him to get better. His wife and he divorced after this event. He becomes agitated when talking about his ex-wife. He has a high school degree and had two years of college and was studying to be a nurse anesthetist when this episode happened. His children live with his ex-wife.

Mr. Abrahamson is a youthful-appearing man who is restless and has a hard time sitting in the office. ... He must have asked the date at least twenty times in a 45 minute interview. His mood and affect was at times cooperative, at times anxious and irritable. At one point when he became agitated and frustrated by my not immediately feeding him the information that he was asking, he stood up, raised his voice and leaned over me in a somewhat threatening manner .... This patient certainly has a significant residual cognitive deficit and would best fall in the category of a diagnosis such as organic brain syndrome. There are some cases noted in which obsessive-compulsive disorder presents following brain injury, and it seems as though he has developed an obsessive-compulsive ritual around asking for information about the date and age. It seems that this might be helped by both a behavioral program as well as some medication. I discussed medication with the family. They had some fears about medication, though by the end of our session were willing to admit that they would try it if it seemed helpful to Gary. ...

Lastly, I think that Gary's parents would benefit from

support and input from the traumatic brain injury team; I believe they have done a fine job but are getting somewhat tired in their efforts and could use some reassuring support and perhaps redirection.

Based on my experience and observations as Gary's caretaker, I took the position that drug therapy never seemed to do much for Gary except, in the short term, sedate him. However, after consulting with the psychiatrist, I agreed to a trial period with Prozac.

Prozac made him more docile and he did seem to sleep slightly better at night, but we soon found out that it also made him urinary incontinent — unable to hold his water. Because of this, the doctor agreed to cut his dosage, and that seemed to help a bit.

Soon after the drug therapy began, the TBI program scheduled Gary to start physical, occupational, and speech therapies. Unfortunately, after three sessions — which went badly — we had to abort the program. Gary became agitated during the therapy sessions. Like before, Gary apparently was threatened by clinical trappings. The therapists seemed generally capable but didn't always use productive techniques for dealing with Gary's perseverative questions. During one session, Gary queried one of the therapists about the date and her age. "We're not here to talk about age," she quickly retorted. At that, Gary became indignant and anxious. Apparently feeling offended, insulted, or provoked, he stood up, shoulders back, and appeared ready to leave. Although the therapy was going fairly well up to that point, the session had to be terminated. Had the therapist simply redirected the conversation away from Gary's favorite subject of year and age, the session could have successfully concluded. Traveling three hours a day for what amounted to twenty to thirty minutes of marginally productive intervention seemed only to confuse and agitate Gary all the more. Another dead end!

In June, Gary's son Arlo graduated from high school. Gary received an invitation — but only after the graduation. Arlo entered the Navy after graduation and in August, after basic training, he visited his father.

About that time, much to my delight, I received a call from Gary's attorney: "We have obtained expert medical opinions. It is their opinion that Gary was the victim of medical malpractice, so we will be filing the lawsuit in Wichita, Kansas

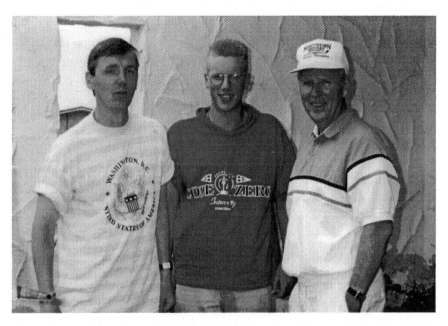

Gary, Arlo (on leave, having just finished Navy basic training), and Gary Sr., 1992.

next week."

What great news! I didn't want to get my hopes up too soon. I tried to maintain a calm exterior despite the excitement I was feeling inside. I had never been involved in a lawsuit before. It would prove to be a tremendous learning experience.

In the fall of 1992, I began my last semester at the University. My class schedule forced me to stay in Marquette two nights a week. I marvelled at my husband's dedication and care of Gary. Truly, without his support and cooperation, I could not have attained my degree.

On December 19, 1992, I graduated as the oldest member of my class. In attendance were all my children and their children — with the sad exception of Arlo and Leif. As I walked across the stage, a voice said: "Patricia Abrahamson, Bachelor of Social Work *cum laude.*" Then came screams, hurrays, and loud applause from my family. What an exhilarating experience.

At the reception later, I was surrounded by my children and grandchildren. Gary congratulated me: "Good job, Mom, I'm proud of you." He attended, he witnessed, he evaluated, he *remembered,* and he responded *so* appropriately. I will remember that day forever!

After graduation, my focus turned to the lawsuit and anticipating how our lives would change if it were successful. A victory would allow Gary to access new, possibly more productive rehabilitative options; it would also guarantee that Gary would continue to be well cared for — even after Gary Senior and I are no longer around.

I looked forward to our day in court.

14

LEGAL MEANS

Litigation is the pursuit of practical ends, not a game of chess.
- Felix Frankfurter

It has been said, somewhat euphemistically, that armed warfare is the pursuit of diplomacy — *by other means*; similarly, the medical malpractice lawsuit was, in part, the pursuit of Gary's future rehabilitative and custodial care — *by other means.*

Not all brain injuries are as debilitating as Gary's. Many, including some caused by a quick blow to the head, are much more mild, more subtle and covert — at least to casual observers. One brain injury victim, a lawyer, experienced a coma for several days before enduring months of recovery. Eventually, he regained the ability to discuss legal issues, help select juries, figure out questions for direct and cross examination, and shape a closing argument. But, for some reason, he could never find the rear entrance to the courtroom each day of trial.

Some brain injuries are even milder than that. A person can have a traumatic brain injury, experts say, even though the victim did not lose consciousness, suffered no skull fracture, was walking and talking after the accident, and scored normal on all diagnostic laboratory tests. Instead, he or she begins to suffer subtle symptoms — minor concentration and attention problems, memory lapses, irritability, anger, frustration, or some difficulty planning or organizing activities. Whereas broken bones are easy to recognize, mild forms of brain injury are not so easily recognized. Therefore, *if* a mild brain injury is successfully identified, and *if* a lawsuit is brought to recover damages from a responsible party, the dominant issue will be *proving* that a compensable brain injury exists.

But proof of a disabling cognitive injury was not a problem in Gary's case; he suffered a severe, not mild, brain injury. The primary issue in Gary's lawsuit would be proving that his brain injury, the result of a heart stoppage, was due to a doctor's misdiagnosis of his heart condition. In other words, a proper diagnosis would have given Gary the opportunity to medically avert (e.g. through medicine and behavioral changes) the tragic consequences of his condition or even surgically rectify (e.g. through heart bypass surgery) his condition. A secondary, yet important, legal issue would be the extent of damages — the appropriate monetary award for his loss of income, his pain and suffering, the cost of future medical, rehabilitative, and custodial care.

As Gary's legal guardian, I was able to initiate the lawsuit on his behalf. Though I had this authority, I didn't have any experience in bringing a lawsuit. The extent of my legal background was limited to movie and television courtroom dramas. I soon found out, however, that many of those portrayals leave out much pre-trial, behind-the-scenes maneuvering.

When the legal process began, I was led to believe that this lawsuit involved only my son. However, in the State of Kansas, an ex-spouse must be notified of the pending suit in order to allow them the opportunity to file a claim for loss of consortium (e.g. loss of companionship and support provided by marriage). So, just months before the trial date, the attorney called me and said, "I've spoken to Kris regarding Gary's suit. As a result, I am filing a claim on her behalf."

At the time, I was shocked and upset at this. I assumed the attorney would represent *only* Gary. To me, this dual representation seemed, potentially, to present a conflict of interest; I feared that an award for Kris *could* mean a smaller amount available for Gary.

The preparatory steps to litigate a medical malpractice suit were extensive and time-consuming. Piles of depositions, interrogatories, and documents were amassed. And because of the technical nature of medicine, an expert witness would be required. In other words, unless the malpractice was, to a layperson, obvious — such as a surgeon leaving a scalpel in someone's stomach after surgery — we needed a doctor willing to testify that Gary's heart stoppage was caused by — or could have been prevented but for — another doctor's medically negligent diagnosis or follow-up.

We also needed other expert witnesses: a vocational economic analyst to determine Gary's lost wages, a medical doctor or neuropsychologist to determine the extent of cognitive damages, a life care planning specialist to determine the cost of his medical, rehabilitative and custodial care, and so on. Then, for every expert witness we found to give favorable testimony, the defense counsel was free to find an expert witness on the same topic to give testimony less favorable to us, more favorable to them.

One of the defense's expert medical witness, Dr. A., spent several hours at our home talking to my husband and me. He spent five minutes with Gary. Gary's lawyer warned us ahead of time that even though Dr. A. may seem to be a nice, caring, congenial man, he is an expert witness for the other side and will not have Gary's best interest in mind. In other words, the lawyer was telling me that even if a pretty, white, and seemingly harmless sheep showed up at our front door, stay guarded — don't let it disarm you; it is a wolf in sheep's clothing.

When the aging, genteel Dr. Wolf-in-Sheep's-Clothing graced our doorstep, one of the first things that rolled off of his long, silvery tongue was an assurance that he was "here in Gary's best interest." We discussed the assertive role that I had taken when Gary's medication seemed to harm, rather than promote, his cognitive and social development. He appeared ever so sympathetic to our cause. He was also helpful, suave, and very good at getting information. When he left, I almost felt guilty for not personally driving this nice, empathetic man to the airport.

Later, when Dr. Wolf-in-Sheep's-Clothing gave a deposition, he stated, "Gary's mother, Patt, has impaired Gary's rehabilitation by refusing to allow Gary to be medicated with various kinds of drugs recommended by his physicians. These medications would make Gary Abrahamson more docile and receptive to rehabilitation, and would decrease the perseveration problem."

At the time, despite the warnings from my lawyer, I was naively baffled: *How could this man agree with me and my position about Haldol and the Tardive dyskinesia it caused in Gary, then make statements directly opposing what was discussed in person? How could this man commend, agree, encourage, and sympathize with me in the presence of Gary's lawyer, my husband, and myself, yet repudiate these positions when it came time to take his deposition?* My stress increased one hundredfold as the trial grew near. I felt that the real issue in this case — damage to Gary caused by the cardiologist's malpractice — became clouded as the defense methodically gathered information intended to distort, confuse, and draw attention toward subsidiary issues.

During the discovery phase of the case, all potential witnesses with even a smidgen of relevant evidence were deposed — including Kris, Gary Senior, Jeff, Vicki, myself, the doctor who treated Gary, expert witnesses on both sides, and so on. Both lawyers usually were physically present for the deposition, which meant scheduling depositions and traveling to several different parts of the country. All of the experts had to be paid for their time.

The process was not only time-consuming but expensive too. We didn't, thank goodness, have to advance this money because attorneys generally take personal injury cases on a contingency fee basis; in other words, the attorney's entire fee is *contingent* upon winning the case. Under that arrangement, Gary owed no legal fees unless and until he was awarded damages — either through a jury verdict or through a settlement agreement. The risk of loss is borne by the attorney. Of course, if there is only a slight chance of winning, the lawyer may not take the case — or at least won't take it on a contingency fee basis. A contingency-fee lawyer will be entitled to somewhere between 25 and 40 percent of proceeds of the case. Most states have a cap on the maximum percentage for contingency fees.

Despite the behind-the-scenes legal machinations leading up to the trial, our overall strategy was relatively straightforward: to present the facts in a light most favorable to our side that would prove by a preponderance of the evidence that Gary's brain injured condition could have been prevented had Gary's cardiologist performed in a manner consistent with the special degree of knowledge ordinarily possessed by other cardiologists.

Assuming we would win on the liability issue, we would also want to emphasize those aspects of Gary's life that would tend to substantiate our claim for damages: his future income lost due to the injury (an amount that would have been enhanced due to his educational pursuits), his medical and therapy bills, and the enormous resources required to care for him the rest of his life.

By contrast, their strategy consisted — at least in part — of digging up evidence that could be used to suggest that Gary was responsible for his own condition. For example, they would likely attempt to confuse the issue by showing that there was a 17-month gap between the time Gary's family doctor recommended he see a cardiologist and the time he actually saw one or by suggesting that Gary failed to provide complete and accurate information about his chest pain and episodes of dizziness and fainting.

As a backup — in the event they would lose on the liability issue — the defense would then want to present the case in such a way as to lower the jury's estimate of damages. They could do this by finding expert witnesses to present the facts in a light most favorable to them (e.g. a vocational economic analyst that would low-ball Gary's expected future earnings, a life care planning specialist that would low-ball the resources needed to care for Gary in the future, and so on).

Though they would be limited by rules that require evidence to be "relevant" to the case, the defense could even try to let the jury in on any negative aspects of Gary's life or any existing dissension within the family. This could help draw the jury's attention away from the merits of the case and make Gary and Kris seem less deserving of sympathy, less worthy of a large award.

Everyone's past life contains some negative elements —

some are evident, some hidden. As the discovery process unfolded, I felt anger, sadness, and hostility. At times I felt my son was a victim all over again as seemingly normal happenings in his life were taken out of context.

The plaintiff builds up the case; the defense tears it down. As the trial date approached I felt drawn into a roller coaster ride I couldn't stop and couldn't control — one day on Cloud Nine, the next thrust into the depths of despair.

Once all of the evidence was gathered, the depositions taken, and the rest of the discovery process completed, our lawyer engaged the services of a firm specializing in trial and jury consulting to help us prepare for the settlement and trial stage of the case.

Trial consultants conduct surveys (e.g., poll people by phone or in person to get a sense of how a cross-section of society would respond to certain arguments), run focus groups (e.g., where five to 15 people are asked what they think about an issue while clients and lawyers either sit in on or record the sessions), and coordinate mock trials to test run the whole case before a mock jury. These simulations are an opportunity to get feedback from disinterested observers.

Using information gathered by the consultants, lawyers are better able to pick effective themes, to anticipate strengths and weaknesses in their case, and to craft opening and closing statements. In short, it helps get you in a position to try the case most effectively.

Sometimes trial consultants are also hired to help attorneys during the jury selection process, which is sometimes referred to as voir dire. The public, somewhat inaccurately, perceives juries as being randomly selected. While it is true that there is an initial random selection from the jury pool, there is an opportunity for lawyers to de-select certain jurors. During the voir dire process, jurors are questioned by either the lawyers or the judge to determine if they hold any biases that could impair their impartiality in a case. The attorneys are then able to de-select jurors for cause (i.e., if a good argument can be made that a potential juror is biased) or by using one of their peremptory challenges (i.e., a certain number of jurors may be de-selected without the need for any stated reason).

In our case, for example, the defense probably would not want a former victim of medical malpractice to sit on the jury; likewise, our side would probably not want a doctor who has been subject — at least in his mind — to frivolous malpractice suits helping to decide the case.

These challenges are intended to produce juries whose collective mind-sets are free of extremes in pre-existing biases. In reality, however, these challenges are used to achieve favorable juries. In order to do that, the lawyers must uncover not only the obvious biases of jurors but the not-so-obvious biases as well.

That is where jury consultants come in. Surveys have suggested that less than ten percent of jurors admit they're leaning one way or the other by the end of voir dire. Jury consultants help attorneys craft questions for voir dire designed to ferret out the truth. They also use psychological profiles or even body language to discern the leanings of potential jurors. For example, since research has suggested that people who touch their noses while speaking may be lying, the consultant can advise the attorneys as to which nefarious nose-touchers to strike.

Though trial consultants have reportedly been used in most of the high-profile cases in the last several years — including trials involving William Kennedy Smith, Heidi Fleiss, Jack Kevorkian, Rodney King, Erik and Lyle Menendez as well as the O.J. Simpson criminal case — they are not just used in high profile or cause célèbre cases. Lawyers are finding them useful in all types of cases, especially when the stakes are high. Some say the profession began in 1971 during the Pennsylvania trial of Daniel and Philip Berrigan, two brothers accused of conspiracy in antiwar activities. Social scientists, sympathetic to the anti-war movement, volunteered to conduct surveys and interviews to help the brothers' defense lawyers pick the juries. Today, trial consultants have backgrounds in psychology, law, sociology, marketing, and survey research methods.

Needless to say, I was amazed at the sophistication of the procedures and the process. I wasn't yet sure if there was a wizard in the field of brain injury, but I *did* learn that there *are* those who claim to be wizards at helping lawyers win cases by emphasizing the right argument and picking the right jurors.

Though it was all very interesting, after a while I simply reached a point where I wished the suit would conclude — that we would settle or go to trial. Of course, while all of this was going on we still had to tend to Gary's needs. During a free moment now and then, I would form a mental image of what the first day of trial might be like.

"Are both sides ready?" the judge asks.

"Yes, your honor," both sides respond.

"Are there any preliminary motions?"

"No, your honor."

"Very well, let's proceed with the opening statements."

Gary's attorney George Grisham (not his real name) walks around his desk, past the judge and stops before the jury box. He clasps his hands together in front of his waist, stares momentarily at the floor to gather his thoughts, and then begins to speak.

Ladies and gentlemen of the jury, counsel, your honor. My name is George Grisham and I, along with my co-counsel Francis Kidd, represent the victim, Gary Abrahamson, Jr., in the case before you today.

On a personal note, in as much as I've always wanted to serve on a jury but was never asked, I must tell you that I have a slight degree of envy for you all. You are sitting here in this courtroom today because you're upstanding citizens of this fine community — nothing more, nothing less. I am here because I went through several years of law studies and spent tens of thousands of dollars in the process. I suspect that you all may have gotten the better end of that deal.

So what's this case all about? This is a case about hopes and dreams — a young man's hopes and dreams that were tragically cut short. Gary Abrahamson's hopes and dreams were dashed when on October 25, 1987, at the young age of 37, he needlessly suffered cardiac arrest; unfortunately, his cardiac arrest, his heart stoppage left him severely brain injured, unable to work, unable to care for himself, unable to function like you and me. I'd now like to introduce you to Gary Abrahamson. Gary could you stand so the jury may know who you are? (Gary stands.) Thank you, Gary — you may sit down.

I am going to take a moment to describe Gary's condition, but first I'd like you all to close your eyes. You just saw Gary but you don't *really* know him yet. So I want you to think of your closest male relative — perhaps your brother, your father, or your son. Now imagine, just imagine, that I am describing not Gary Abrahamson, a man you don't yet know, but your closest male relative. What if *he* — that vital, caring and intelligent person you love — is suddenly brain injured; what if *he* suffers from severe memory loss; *he* is unable to engage in goal-directed behavior or plan for the future; *he* is confused, disoriented, lacks insight, and has difficulty sleeping; *he* is unable to independently dress himself; *he* is unable to independently bathe himself; *he* lacks all bladder control while sleeping and you must put a diaper on him, or if that is below his dignity you must be prepared to wash him, change his underwear and sheets at 1:00 a.m., and then again at 6:00 a.m.; *he* is unable to independently feed himself; *he* is unable to return to work or gainful employment; *he* requires 24-hour supervision.

What a horror. But, you say, at least he is still alive, at least he is still here to talk to and have a relationship with. Then you find out that you can't talk to him — or at least you can't talk to him like you used to — for he is no longer the same person. In fact, he is a stranger. He is unable to control his emotions; he is unable to carry on a normal conversation; he asks you the same questions 100, maybe 200 times a day: "What year is this? How old am I? How old are you?" And when you answer, he accuses you of lying; he is unable to remember what happened yesterday, or even earlier the same day; he makes socially inappropriate statements; he is severely brain damaged and will not fully recover.

You may open your eyes. Someone once said that the truth will make you free — but first it will make you miserable. Well, ladies and gentlemen of the jury, the truth of this case, as the evidence will show, is that Gary Abrahamson (pointing at Gary) placed his trust in a medical specialist, the defendant Dr. Z. (pointing at the defendant), and suffered debilitating and tragic consequences.

But you know, Gary wasn't always this way. Gary used to be just like many of us. Like most, Gary wasn't rich; he wasn't famous; he wasn't even powerful. Yet he had a bright future ahead of him. He was a man with a wonderful family — a beautiful wife Kristine and two lovely boys, Arlo and Leif; a man who grew up in Michigan but came to this great State of Kansas in 1982 to pursue work and set down new roots for his young family; a man whose family adjusted well to their new community in Great Bend, who made many new friends at the local Baptist church they attended; a man who married young, who got a late start on his education, but in his mid-30's had recently received his associate's degree and was studying to be a nurse; a man with a tremendous potential to bring happiness and prosperity to himself and his family.

But Gary was never able to realize his potential or carry out his dreams. And for Gary's family, those dreams have been replaced with sadness, anger, and grief. Gary's handicap left him unable to support his wife, unable to nurture his children. Like a thief in the night, Gary's brain injury snatched both normalcy and happiness from Gary's family. Eventually, Gary's family broke apart. As often happens in these cases, the duties of parenthood, the obligation of 24-hour care, the responsibility of managing a household, and the difficulties of caring for a dependent, sometimes hostile and bewildering brain injured spouse became overwhelming. Within two years of his cardiac arrest, Gary had lost his spouse and his children. Today, Gary Abrahamson, after 17 years of marriage, a man in his forties, lives — out of necessity — with his parents. And although Gary has memory loss, he has not forgotten his family. Gary often tells his parents, "I've lost my wife, my kids, my job, my life, and everything." Despite his severe brain injury, he *is* cognizant of his losses.

So what happened? What went tragically wrong for Gary and his young family? After all, Gary was a well-conditioned athlete; he watched his weight; he occasionally lifted weights; he regularly jogged five miles a day. Why did Gary suffer cardiac arrest at 37 years old?

The answer to what went wrong, the evidence will show, can be traced directly to Gary's doctor visits in the several months leading up to his cardiac arrest. In July 1985, Gary's family doctor recommended that he have a treadmill stress test. This test, which records a patient's heart rhythm using an electrocardiogram while the patient is exercised on a treadmill, may be used by a doctor to determine if there are any abnormalities that may suggest the presence of coronary artery disease. Because the test *did* show some irregularities that suggested the presence of coronary artery disease, Gary's family doctor referred him to Dr. Z., a cardiologist, who is a specialist in diagnosing and treating heart-related problems — precisely the type of medical specialist that could have likely prevented Gary's cardiac arrest.

In December 1986, when Gary stepped into the defendant's office, he had no reason not to put his full trust in Dr. Z., the heart specialist. On that day, Dr. Z. examined Gary and evaluated his abnormal treadmill stress test results, and then made a diagnosis. The evidence will show that Dr. Z.'s diagnosis all but sealed Gary's fate that day; in short, Dr. Z. concluded that Gary *did not* have coronary artery disease; rather, the stress test irregularity was, Dr. Z. concluded, due to mitral valve prolapse — a mere heart valve problem. He told Gary not to worry, that the heart valve condition wouldn't cause him any problems, and to continue his regime of jogging five miles daily. Dr. Z. decided, without the benefit of conducting any other tests, that Gary's treadmill stress test *did not* indicate the presence of coronary artery disease; rather, he concluded, the stress test was a false-positive test; there was no coronary artery disease — only a harmless valve condition.

Now, you're going to hear a lot of evidence in this case, including expert medical witnesses on both sides. After carefully and honestly evaluating the evidence, you will need to determine whether Dr. Z. was negligent; after carefully and honestly evaluating the evidence, you will need to determine whether Gary's brain injury could have been prevented. And after hearing both sides, I think you will come to agree that Dr. Z. was wrong about the stress test being false-positive. Although it was later confirmed by a different doctor that Gary *did* have a mild mitral valve prolapse, the valve condition was *not* the major diagnostic dilemma that Dr. Z. was obligated to identify; in fact, the evidence will show that Gary *did* have severe coronary artery disease when Dr. Z. examined him; the evidence will show that Dr. Z. failed to obtain a complete and accurate medical history of Gary related to possible coronary artery disease; the evidence will show that — given Gary's irregular stress test results, his family history of heart disease, his elevated cholesterol level, his male gender, and his chest pain syndrome, all of which Dr. Z. knew or should have known — Dr. Z. should *not* have ruled out coronary disease; the evidence will show that Dr. Z.'s reasons for dismissing the positive stress test as a false-positive could be explained by Gary's excellent physical condition; the evidence will show that, under the circumstances, it was negligent for Dr. Z. to use mitral valve prolapse to explain the abnormal stress test without doing further tests to confirm his preliminary conclusion; the evidence will show that if Dr. Z. *had* conducted these tests, he would have confirmed that Gary *did* have coronary artery disease; the evidence will show that Gary's cardiac arrest — which came a mere 9 months, 23 days after Dr. Z. examined Gary — *was* the result of coronary artery disease; the evidence will show that had a proper diagnosis been made, had Dr. Z. not so quickly ruled out the existence of coronary artery disease, that Gary's cardiac arrest and resulting brain damage could have been prevented.

As you evaluate whether the defendant was negligent in making an evaluation of Gary Abrahamson's condition on December 2, 1986, I want you to recognize that Dr. Z. held Gary's life in his hands; Dr. Z. wasn't simply charged with hooking up cable TV to someone's house, or diagnosing why a garbage disposal doesn't work, or providing advice about whether an air conditioner should be replaced. Dr. Z. was dealing with someone's life; Gary was depending upon him; Gary's wife was depending upon him; Gary's children were depending upon him; even Gary's grandchildren — yet unborn — will be affected by Dr. Z.'s negligence.

But, be prepared. The defense is going to try to confuse the issue of whether Dr. Z. was negligent. They will try to shift the focus away from Dr. Z.'s negligence. Listen to their argument, then systematically and critically analyze it, but always keep in mind — always weigh their arguments against — the duty that Dr. Z. owed to his patient Gary Abrahamson.

First, the defense may point to a 17-month interval from the time that Gary was first advised to see a cardiologist and the time when he did see Dr. Z. I could tell you that Kris was working two part-time jobs and Gary was in school: that during this time period, they did not have medical insurance: that as soon as one of them resumed a full-time job and medical insurance was in place, Gary wasted little time in making the appointment with a cardiologist. I could offer that as an explanation. Instead, however, I am going to suggest to you that this 17-month interval is simply a red herring — it's irrelevant to the allocation of legal liability in this case. While waiting the 17 months was not smart, the evidence will show that no injury resulted. And the fact remains that Dr. Z. had the last clear chance to discover Gary's condition and thereby prevent Gary's cardiac arrest and resulting brain injury.

Let me give you my smoke detector analogy. Think of Gary's 17-month delay as though he lived in his house without a smoke detector for an equivalent period; no fire occurs during that 17-month period; at the end of the 17-month period, Gary installs a smoke detector. Some months later, the house catches on fire; because it had been defectively manufactured, the smoke detector fails to go off; the house burns down with Gary inside, and he is injured. The company that defectively manufactured the smoke detector may be liable for Gary's injuries; Gary's 17-month delay in installing the smoke detector wasn't smart; he subjected himself to risk during that 17 months — no doubt about it. But, there was no fire during the 17 months that Gary went without a smoke detector. The bottom line is this: the company that defectively manufactured the smoke detector may not, logically, defend itself by pointing out that Gary waited 17 months to install it. It's irrelevant. And so too is the 17-month interval in the case before you today — it is irrelevant to the issue of whether Dr. Z. was negligent. It is an improper basis on which to shift the blame. The real significance of the number 17 in this case before you lies in the fact that Gary's marriage lasted about 17 years before his brain injured condition — which could have been prevented — brought it to an unhappy end.

Next, the defense may attempt to confuse the liability issue by suggesting that Gary didn't use common sense, that he didn't heed the warning signs; they may contend that Gary should have discontinued his exercise regime and gotten re-evaluated after the December 2, 1986 appointment with Dr. Z., when he experienced additional episodes of chest pain. If Gary continued to run five miles daily after his appointment with Dr. Z. — and he did — he did so because Dr. Z. reassured Gary that it was all right. Dr. Z. reassured Gary that his chest pains were merely the result of the heart valve condition. He reassured Gary that the heart valve condition was benign, unhazardous, and harmless. Gary, a mere layman, untrained in medicine, had absolutely no rational basis on which to dispute, contradict, or challenge Dr. Z.'s diagnosis and advice. Gary continued to run because Dr. Z., the person Gary was relying on for expert medical advice, told him it was OK for him to run.

Let me quickly point out something else. Gary followed an exercise regime *not* because he wanted to take unwarranted risks with his body or because he was a running fanatic willing to go for his daily jog no matter what the cost. Gary ran, in part, because it made him feel better, and he knew that it would strengthen his heart. Gary was well aware of the history of heart disease in his family. So when you think of Gary's running regime, don't think of Gary, the risk-taker: quite the contrary. Eating right, watching his weight, and exercising was a way that he could increase his chances of living a long, healthy life.

Before I leave the liability issue and briefly discuss the issue of damages, I want to again emphasize that whatever the defense tries to throw at you to confuse the issue of who is liable, please consider it against the overwhelming evidence to the contrary, and keep firmly in mind the duty that Dr. Z. owed to his patient Gary Abrahamson. *Don't* let them succeed in getting you to focus on subsidiary or irrelevant issues.

Now, if you *do* conclude that Dr. Z. was negligent and therefore liable, you will need to decide the appropriate measure of damages for Gary and Kris. Gary's damages include past and future medical care and therapy, lost wages due to his inability to work, past and future expenses to maintain around-the-clock custodial care for him until he dies, as well as compensation for his pain, suffering, mental anguish, and quality-of-life losses. Kris, Gary's wife at the time of his cardiac arrest, is legally entitled to damages for loss of consortium — her loss of companionship, affection, and emotional and financial support.

With regard to the amount of damages, I won't discuss them in detail in this opening statement other than to say that you will hear from several expert witnesses. You will hear from a vocational economic analyst to determine Gary's lost wages. You will also hear from a lifecare planner, a rehabilitation consultant, and an economist to estimate the amount of money it will cost to provide Gary humane care — medical, rehabilitative, therapeutic, and custodial — for the remainder of his life.

Again, you will hear conflicting testimony. What I want you to be aware of here is that the defense will likely pursue a two-pronged strategy: Number one, they will argue that Dr. Z. was not negligent in his treatment of Gary; or if he was negligent, it was not the proximate cause of Gary's damages. If you don't buy either of these arguments — and you are not likely to after you've heard the evidence — the defense will then try to get you to minimize your estimation of damages. Gary's expert witnesses will estimate Gary's lost wages and the cost of his care as well as his life expectancy. The defense witnesses will then testify to a lower amount for each of these items.

In addition, the defense may try to play on your sympathies — or your lack of sympathies. For example, in order to minimize the damages you provide for Kris for loss of consortium, the defense may point out that Kris left Gary and is now divorced; they may suggest that Kris walked away from the problems and made a life for herself; the implicit message here is that you should, therefore, minimize the amount of damages you provide for her loss of consortium. Let me first suggest that Gary's brain injured condition is not Kris' fault. Let me also suggest that if the defense does pursue this tactic, they probably won't mention that as a result of Gary's brain injury, Kris quit her job and temporarily abandoned her career, that Kris was forced to abandon the Kansas community which her family had come to esteem; the defense probably won't emphasize that Kris lost her marriage, that the children lost their father, that they all lost Gary's financial and emotional support; the defense won't want you to focus on the fact that Kris gave up time with her sons to care for Gary, that she lost a husband, a friend, and companion in the process, that she is left without the person she married, that her kids will not grow up with the love and support of their dad, that in many ways she had to start over with only memories of their former life together. Listen to all of the evidence, and I think you will conclude that there was enough pain, suffering, and emotional distress to go around and that Kris did the best she could under the circumstances.

Finally, let me say just a couple of words about Gary's current caretakers, his parents. Gary's mother and father — who are responsible for Gary's around-the-clock care, who are attempting to cope under trying circumstances,

who generally refrain from taking Gary to normal social
events because when he sees other people, normal people,
he gets anxious and frustrated at the heightened realization that he's not normal, sometimes sparking outbursts
— they essentially have had to give up a normal life in order to accommodate Gary's life. But Gary's aging parents
won't be around forever and Gary may outlive his parents
by a significant number of years. The damages you award
Gary will not only pay for his past and current medical,
rehabilitative, and other care, but it will also be used to
assure that he continues to have humane care once his
parents are no longer around. Let me assure you that
whatever the amount of damages you decide to award to
Gary Abrahamson, all of these funds will be placed in a
special account that will be supervised by the probate court
throughout the remainder of his life.

Thank you.*

That is what I imagined Gary's lawyer might say in an
opening statement at trial. The trial date, set for September of
1993, still seemed to be well off in the distance, but fast approaching. Closing in on us even faster was the settlement
conference. Set one month before trial, the settlement conference was intended to provide a forum — after all of the evidence had been gathered — for a final attempt to settle the
case, thereby avoiding the necessity of a full-blown trial.

By July 1993, the whole process was becoming a thorn in
my side as we attempted to effectively advocate for Gary *and*
continue to meet his physical, psychological, and developmental needs.

---

* This opening statement you have just read did not really occur. The case settled and never actually went to trial. This fictitious
opening statement is based, in part, on opinions provided at pre-
trial depositions by Gary's expert medical witnesses. The reader
should know, of course, that Dr. Z's (which by the way is not his real
initial) expert medical witnesses gave contrary opinions in pre-trial
depositions. Therefore, the fictitious opening statement should not
be taken by the reader as the author's statement of fact; it consti-
tutes the author's opinion of what a lawyer representing the plain-
tiffs might have said had the case gone to trial.

Before the settlement conference, we all agreed before-hand on what percentage Gary and Kris would each receive from an overall award. This allowed us to work together during the settlement negotiations, enabling our lawyer to ethically represent both of our interests, toward the common goal of achieving as large an overall settlement award for Gary and Kris as possible.

I left for Wichita, where the conference was to take place, in August of 1993. The tremendous responsibility weighed heavily on me. Questions plagued me throughout the flight, circling in my mind like a plane waiting for a runway. *What would a fair settlement amount to? Should we even consider any settlement? How will I react when I stand face to face with the doctor whom we believe to be responsible for massive changes in all our lives? What if we go to trial? Will I be able to stand up to the denigrations and exaggerations posed by the defense attorney? Could Gary be harmed by the lawyer's dual representation at trial of both Kris and Gary? What if I don't accept a settlement and Gary loses the lawsuit?* All these decisions would have a profound effect on the rest of Gary's life!

I arrived in Wichita late in the afternoon and took a taxi to the hotel. The plan was to meet with Gary's attorney that evening for last minute briefings and to get an update before the conference, scheduled for the next day.

The stress was enormous. Gary's lawyer informed me as to the amount of the doctor's medical malpractice insurance limit. Unfortunately, the clinic, where the doctor worked, also had an obligation to provide more insurance but had negligently let the policy lapse. He also informed me that, in case of a settlement, the proceeds would come in ten annual installments.

My head was spinning. *How will this lawsuit play out? Settlement? Trial? Win? Lose?* The night before the settlement conference, I tossed and turned. In the morning I felt sick, headachy, and shaky.

We arrived at the huge office complex downtown which housed the defense attorney's law firm. Gary's lawyer, an associate lawyer, and I were escorted to a gigantic conference room. Gary's lawyer gave me last-minute instructions: "Remember, Patt, don't show any non-verbals in facial expres-

sions — no frowns, no surprises, no stares, no emotion, nothing."

My head pounded as a large number of men dressed in
dark suits and ties filed into the room. The only other woman
present was an associate attorney with the defense counsel.

I whispered to our lawyer: "Which one is the doctor?"

"He's directly across from you," he answered, not lifting
his head in that direction. The table must have been 20 feet
across.

Silence prevailed as the mediator began. "I will be meeting privately with both the defense and the plaintiff in an effort to reach an agreement. I have been presented with a
synopsis from each lawyer regarding this case. At the end of
the process, I will give you my opinion as to which side will be
successful if this case goes to trial. Each lawyer may now
present their case."

Gary's lawyer spoke first. His stalwart performance was
delivered articulately and eloquently. His summation was
strong as he presented a synopsis of our case, including testimony from expert witnesses. He also pointed out several statements from one of the defense expert witnesses which actually helped our case. "The defendant Dr. Z. is articulate, with
good presence. And so is Gary's mother and the family I'm
representing — so that's a wash." Again, I was amazed at the
detailed considerations. *Everything* is weighed as to the projected response of the jury.

I felt confident as I listened to his presentation — until,
that is, the defense presented their case. At one point, defense counsel addressed me personally: "Mrs. Abrahamson,
you are aware that a settlement is a compromise on both parts?
I'm going to show that your son ignored his health and verify
that he did not even tell you, his parents, about his condition.
He wanted to run at any expense. He neglected to tell the
doctor all the facts surrounding his chest pain."

I sat mute, fighting an urge to cry out: *That's not true! He
is twisting the facts! Gary had called us worried about his
health. He had informed us about the impending tests. He
had informed us of the results — and yes, he had received a
clean bill of health, along with encouragement to continue his
running. Yes, it was true he loved to run, but it wasn't the way*

he was describing it at all.

As I fought my emotions, I worried that they might transform my facial expressions and speak louder than words — something my lawyer had forewarned me against. Defense counsel concluded by saying, "If we go to trial, you can count on an appeal: remember, that can hold up everything a year or two, maybe longer."

After the summary statements, we returned to our separate conference rooms. The mediator met with our side first. "After reviewing both sides, my feeling is that you have a stronger case and should win if you go to trial." He told us he thought he could get the defense to settle for the full amount of the doctor's insurance monies available. I wanted to sign on the dotted line and run. But my lawyer was not satisfied; he put in a bid for additional settlement money that would be paid by the clinic, which had failed to keep up their insurance policy but was still potentially liable in this case.

The mediator stepped in: "I don't think we'll be able to do that: the clinic has financial problems ..." And so it went, the mediator shuffling back and forth between the two sides that were separated only by another conference room.

We didn't settle then. The full amount of the doctor's malpractice insurance monies was on the table, but the clinic representatives said they had to have a board meeting to determine whether they would be willing to settle for the amount we were asking.

My lawyer wanted to go to trial; he was willing to take the risk that we would do as well or better. Besides that, I believe he hadn't had a full-blown trial in about two years and may have been itching to have one. By contrast, I was inclined to settle. How could I gamble Gary's future? Gary could receive a sizeable amount of money now or possibly *nothing* if we went to trial.

I left for home that evening, uneasy and anxious about waiting the three days it would take for the clinic's board to meet. A few days later, Gary's lawyer called: "Apparently, the clinic board attempted to meet but wasn't able to muster a quorum," he said. "Therefore, there still has been no consideration of the issue and the board doesn't have another meeting scheduled for another two weeks." Meanwhile, the trial date was closing in fast — in about three weeks. My lawyer advised me that, since we had not yet agreed to settle and since the board would not meet for another two weeks, the other side — by necessity — was preparing for trial. He also stated that there was a remote possibility that they would decide to withdraw their offer. After some further discussion, I made a command decision: "I want to settle for the full amount of the doctor's insurance policy as had been proposed."

"Patt, I'd love to go to trial, but I understand your position and what you are going through," he responded. "I'll call the defense attorney and inform them of your decision, then I'll call you back after I reach him."

Two weeks later, I took another flight to Kansas. I appeared before the judge and everything was signed and sealed. Gary realized about half of the total settlement amount after attorney's fees, expenses, and the agreed-upon amount for his ex-wife. Although it's a large amount, it may not be enough to pay for all of Gary's care and treatment for the rest of his life — that figure was projected somewhat in excess of what we were able to get for him. My feeling of relief, however, was profound. Thank goodness it was over and successful. Now, Gary would have funds available for treatments and therapy and his future care would be fairly secure. He would not be disabled and indigent, dependent upon the state for his care.

Although the case never went before an actual jury, the mock trial conducted by the trial consultants produced a litany of responses.

One of the questions posed to the mock jury was whether my decision to extend Gary's life with bypass surgery would effect their decision about whether or not Dr. Z. is liable for Gary's injuries or damages. They responded as follows:

- I believe Gary's mother's reasoning was clouded by her love for her son.
- The mother acted in good faith.
- This is a personal, not legal, principal — it has no bearing on this case.
- The doctor is liable no matter how long Gary lives.
- I believe she made an intolerable situation even more

unbearable by extending his life.
- The damage was done before the bypass surgery.
- I just consider it a mother's right to extend her son's life — I don't want to question the consequences of her decision.

Comments from the mock jurors about the overall case were just as varied. When asked what this case is all about, they responded as follows:

- A man whose medical condition was not correctly diagnosed by his doctor.
- A young man who maintained his fitness by running and other exercises but had a dangerous heart condition that went undetected by a heart specialist. The man was told he had minor problems, not to worry, and to continue running. The doctor was aware of medical history and test results indicating a problem. The doctor failed to provide reasonable medical care and advice to the young man who, after having a heart attack, suffered severe brain damage.
- A young man who was partly to blame because he exercised excessively despite his family medical history; medical malpractice on the part of a doctor resulting in a dysfunctional life for Gary and his family.
- A doctor's failure to take the time and effort to ensure the well-being of his patient, who became a victim. The doctor is supposedly the expert upon whose reliance we can depend. The doctor failed in his responsibility.
- A young man with a wife and two sons, concerned about good health through exercise, who followed expert medical guidance, and had a heart attack, which resulted in severe brain damage, disruption of lives, and loss of family.
- A family man who, in his zeal to exercise, ignored danger signs he should have heeded and as a consequence caused misery and suffering for many and of a doctor who had the misfortune to examine him.
- Greed.
- A tragic incident in one family's life that was probably

going to happen anyway given the family history, life-style choices, etc., regardless of Dr. Z.'s treatment in 1986. Bypass surgery did not seem warranted then.

- A tragedy in a family caused by some stupid moves on Gary's part, an incomplete duty of Dr. Z., a bad decision by Gary's mother (to have bypass surgery), and not enough push for tests by Kris.
- A young man with a history of heart disease in his family, whose doctor was very negligent in diagnosing his case leaving the young man a brain damaged, helpless person.
- Story of a young man who was driven by the need to exercise and failed to consider his heart problems.
- The negligence and malpractice of Dr. Z. He failed to perform his duties as a specialist, which resulted in brain damage of a patient.
- Sick man, has no wife or family, needs lots of money to live.
- A tragic accident that was not entirely anyone's fault and a family trying to receive payment from the doctor.
- People who made decisions that should have been made only when every possible method of diagnosis, treatment, etc., had been taken.
- A doctor's negligence and a patient's inattentiveness to his own body signals and his blind faith in the doctor's advice to continue his normal activity.
- Malpractice caused by a doctor that should be put out of business if all of his patients are treated that way.
- A medical malpractice suit involving a 37-year-old man who suffered a cardiac arrest while jogging subsequent to a visit to a heart specialist who had assured him that he did not have heart disease and should continue to jog and exercise as before.
- A young man who proceeded to live without heeding the warning signs of past health history, etc., and doctors who didn't take the time to delve beyond the surface and the worst case scenario that resulted.
- A man and his family who are suffering the effects of an unfortunate accident which may have been prevented by

better patient-doctor communication.

- A family who should have known better. A doctor not taking proper tests. A bad decision having bypass surgery.
- The negligence of a doctor and the failure of a family to recognize this and pull together for the patient's benefit.
- A man who could have led a normal life if he had used common sense in his lifestyle. The brain damage he experienced caused his family to disintegrate, incur much expense, and suffer much heartache.
- A person who did not assume responsibility for himself, a doctor who did not provide adequate follow-up, and a family which is greedy.
- An average man with a heart disease which was not properly diagnosed. He died and was revived, only to be brain damaged for life. He was damaged due to negligence of a doctor. His family (wife, children and parents) will suffer for years.
- A family whose life was torn apart because of the sudden and unexpected disease of a family member. This disease will cause a lifetime of sadness, lifestyle change, and expenses.
- A person who had a cardiac arrest, a doctor who did his very best, and a family suffering with all the problems of a brain damaged adult.
- A man with a history of heart disease on both sides of his family, who waited 17 months to see a cardiologist. Ten months after the cardiologist assured him he was fine, he suffered a cardiac arrest and irreparable brain damage.
- Tragedy striking a family and testing their ability to cope. Everyone involved should take some responsibility. Money, however, will not cure Gary or make any of the pain and suffering go away. This family needs to move on with their lives and try to heal themselves the best way they can. Use the money awarded and his social security payments and other government money to place him in a home where he can be handled by professionals.
- A man with a family history of heart disease, who did not

take his symptoms seriously, and a doctor who didn't take them seriously either.

- A family torn apart by the trauma of a loved one with serious brain damage that could conceivably been avoided by a proper diagnosis.
- A young man who was given shallow advice from an expert medical professional, who is now no longer competent to take care of himself or the family he helped create.
- Mother and son fighting for the right things to be done for her son.
- Doctor's lack of interest in patient testing. Patient not following up on health care. Patient loses his family. Has to rely on aging parents.

Had the case gone to trial, my guess is that Gary would have prevailed. That said, however, it *does* appear that the jurors would have had some lively discussion before reaching any conclusions!

15

STILL SEARCHING

There is only one cardinal rule:
One must always listen to the patient.
                                        - Dr. Oliver Sacks

Shortly before Gary's lawsuit was settled, I made arrangements with a well-known rehabilitation facility in Chicago. I read that this institution was one of the ten best rehabilitation facilities in the nation. I wanted to be ready to go forward with Gary's rehabilitation needs if the lawsuit was successful. I wanted direction from the best.

In some cognitive areas, Gary was slowly reclaiming his abilities; there were improvements in vocabulary, spelling, memory, and ability to quickly calculate math problems. Behaviorally, however, Gary had regressed; his perseverative tendencies to pinch, poke, and repeat questions increased.

I needed so many questions answered. Which facilities focused primarily on behavioral programs for individuals with a brain injury? What was Gary's prognosis for continuing improvement? Could *anyone* help his perseveration problem? I was willing to go anywhere in the country for any length of time. I just needed some concrete answers — some direction.

Like Dorothy in the *Wizard of Oz*, I yearned for the good old days, a restoration of life — Gary's life — as it had been in Kansas, before this bad dream began. Like the scarecrow, Dorothy's friend in need of a brain, Gary *also* needed increased cognitive abilities. I hoped and prayed for the existence of a wizard — some person or institution that could rescue Gary from the abyss. All we needed to do, I imagined, was to find the yellow brick road; such a path would lead us to Emerald City, where we would find the wizard, Gary's secular savior.

Our first stop was Chicago, a six-hour drive from our home in Escanaba. We arrived a day in advance of Gary's scheduled appointment because we wanted to get a good night's sleep before the evaluations.

I had made the appointment months in advance and forwarded tons of Gary's medical records. In the morning, Gary seemed rested and relaxed as we walked from our nearby hotel to the rehabilitation facility to begin a new series of evaluations.

His first appointment was with a physician. The examination was fairly routine, something that Gary had been through numerous times since his cardiac arrest. At the close of this meeting, the doctor suggested perhaps a trial of L-Dopa might be in order.

The next scheduled evaluation was with the occupational therapist, set for after lunch. We sat patiently waiting for almost an hour after the set appointment time. Gary soon became restless. In turn, I became concerned that his performance would suffer; I was trying to control any variables that might alter test results. I approached the desk.

"How late are the appointments running?" I asked.

"What's his name again?" the receptionist asked.

"Gary Abrahamson," I replied.

"We don't have an appointment for Gary on the roster," she said. "Are you sure this is the right day and time?"

Exasperated, I fumbled through the papers I had brought.

"Here's my letter confirming the appointment," I said, somewhat indignant.

"I'm going to have to make some calls," she responded. "Don't worry — we'll get it straightened out."

"I *am* worried," I said. "We're from Upper Michigan, and we've waited months for this appointment!"

A short time later, they found a therapist who could evaluate Gary. Once in the room with her, I asked, "What about all the medical records I sent in advance? Have you seen them?"

"No," she responded, "but we've requested that those records be sent up to this floor."

I could feel myself losing patience, losing tolerance. I felt as if we were mere objects, with no one in charge, no one really interested. They spent a lot of time apologizing, but that did little to change my impression. I gazed at all the people lined up in wheelchairs, holding their records. The scene resembled some kind of mass production assembly line, not a human services situation.

In her report, the occupational therapist noted that she would "provide family with recommendations for home management and follow through of additional tasks at home" as well as refer us to possible day programs in our home state to provide structure and to work on orientation and social skills. There was never any follow-up — we were never given such information.

Next, we went to see the physical therapist. Again, he had not reviewed the records in advance. Much of the time was spent answering questions about Gary's background and status before the substantive evaluation began.

That evening, we went back to the hotel, feeling disappointed and discouraged.

The next day, our first appointment was with the speech therapist. She was an excellent clinician. She immediately recognized Gary's apprehensive reaction to clinical environments; to make Gary feel as comfortable as possible, she asked Gary Senior and me to sit in on the evaluation and testing.

She made the following observations, among others:

> Functionally, the patient demonstrated comprehension of simple conversation with repetition and/or restatement. Difficulty with memory and attention as well as low frustration tolerance interferes.
>
> In the area of oral expression, the patient demonstrated the ability to inconsistently express his basic needs. Perseveration and accelerated speech rate as well as sudden increases in intensity were also observed. Reduced initiation of purposeful speech was noted. In the area of reading comprehension, the patient demonstrated the ability to comprehend at the sentence level. Low frustration tolerance, memory and attention may interfere as the length and complexity of reading material increases.
>
> In the area of written expression, the patient demonstrated the ability to convey his ideas through writing. Reduced legibility was noted due to the increased rate. The

patient appeared to be able to follow verbal instructions to slow his writing and speaking rate.

In the area of proprieties, the patient demonstrated inappropriate touching behavior, which appeared to increase when brought to his attention. Redirection ... appeared to reduce this behavior. Perseverative questioning also interfered with the communication process. The patient's frustration increased if his perseverative questions were not addressed ... In the area of written expression, the patient demonstrated the ability to write words to dictation accurately. He also demonstrated the ability to write a narrative consisting of simple sentences with connected ideas. Again, reduced attention and frustration interfered. ...

Positive factors include Gary's use of compensating strategies for orientation to day, date, and time and his ability to increase task orientation following redirection. Recommendations: (1) improve attention and concentration; (2) decrease perseverative speech and behaviors (3) increase initiation for self-help, verbally and in writing; (4) increase structure in daily environment; (5) increase interaction within his familiar community; (6) a structured day treatment program to address the above goals; (7) results of this evaluation were discussed with the patient's parents. The prognosis for improvement is fair to good with treatment. Positive factors include patient's ability to be re-directed. Negative factors include varying frustration levels, memory, and attention. No treatment indicated (because) patient lives out of state. A structured day treatment program near the patient's familiar environment is recommended. The family will be given some suggestions on providing more structure in Gary's environment to improve his skills.

I thought her report was right on target. I was, however, again disappointed that we were never given the follow-up suggestions promised in her report.

In general, I have found that therapists are good — at least on paper — at evaluations and recommendations. For instance, she recommended that Gary decrease perseverative speech and behaviors. But, then again, I didn't need to drive to Chicago for that recommendation. I knew that. Gary's previous medical records indicated that. What I needed to know was where we can go for help and what can be done to facilitate improvement. I needed concrete answers, remedial therapies, specific programs — not generalizations and mere descriptions of the problem.

At this point, we had one more appointment left. This was an important one: an evaluation by the neuropsychologist. We were informed at the central desk that this evaluation would take several hours.

A young assistant came to escort Gary to this appointment. We retreated to the cafeteria for coffee and a snack. Two hours later, we returned to the floor where Gary was being tested, thinking we would still have hours to wait.

The receptionist, appearing concerned, approached us.

"Are you the Abrahamsons?" she asked.

"Yes, we are," I replied.

"Dr. B. would like to speak to you right away," she said.

"Is something wrong?" I asked sensing the urgency in her manner.

"Your son has been taken to the psychiatric floor," she said.

"What happened?" I asked.

"He is being monitored by an aide there," she said. "The doctor will explain." Puzzled and concerned, I waited for the doctor.

Soon, a young, pleasant-appearing man approached us.

"I'm Dr. B." he said, shaking my hand. "We were unable to test Gary due to his perseverative poking and touching behavior."

"I don't understand," I said. "He's been evaluated without incident by other therapists — just yesterday by a speech pathologist."

"Gary touched my assistant's behind, and poked me as he questioned my age and his age," he said. "I told him his behavior was inappropriate, and he became more insistent in poking."

As the doctor was explaining the situation, my mind began to focus. *No wonder he had problems,* I thought. *When you reprimand or focus on inappropriate behavior, it increases. That's why we use the ignore-and-redirect approach. It works. But why isn't this clinician aware of this? Surely he deals with this every day. The speech pathologist had just agreed that redirecting Gary in such situations is the best approach.*

The doctor directed my husband to the floor where Gary was detained. I followed the doctor to his office for more in-depth discussion concerning Gary. I mentioned the L-Dopa treatment suggested by the first physician. His response: "Gary would go right through the ceiling with that drug," contradicting what the other doctor had said.

I asked the doctor where I could get behavioral treatment for Gary. "I have a colleague who works for HealthSouth in St. Louis. I understand they have a good behavioral program. There's another one in Texas. I'll have to get the name and forward it to you."

I thought: *That's it?! No specific directions? No authoritative list of recommended facilities for specific problems? That's all we're doing — spending more time and effort on evaluation, which could be added to the long list of evaluations in my file cabinet at home?*

Later, I got a copy of the neuropsychologist's report. He made several observations, including the following:

> Unfortunately, the patient [acted] in a manner that precluded extensive testing (or testing that would have yielded valid or useful results). Although fully alert and displaying fluent speech as well as intact comprehension for conversational speech and simple commands, he was extremely perseverative, displayed inappropriate touching behavior, and showed severe short-term memory deficit ... He was disoriented to time and place, was very distractible, and often stood up and attempted to leave the room for no apparent reason. Following each question, he responded "Why?;" during periods of conversation, he repeatedly asked questions such as "How old are you?" and "Do you like me?," or made statements such as "I lost my wife and my job." After we answered his questions several times, he could not recall our response. His speech was rapid making it unintelligible at times. Probably the most difficult aspect of his presentation was inappropriate touching. He patted the female examiner on the buttocks several times, and kept poking me in the thigh or ribs when speaking. He was told to discontinue this [and provided a reason when he asked why he should discontinue it] but did not stop.
> ... At the time of his cardiac arrest, he was preparing to become a nurse-anesthetist ... He presently lives with his

parents. His mother has become very involved in his care and has become very educated about neurobehavioral disturbances after brain insults. She noted that he currently has someone work with him for 5 1/2 hours per day on various activities. He also works on a personal computer about 6 hours per week on activities such as writing letters.

According to his mother, some facets of his condition have declined over the past 18-24 months despite the fact that he otherwise made considerable progress in other areas. For example, his articulation is now worse; the perseveration is considerably worse, and the inappropriate touching only began during the past two years ... Mrs. Abrahamson describes her son as someone who was "a little macho before who is now probably very sexually frustrated." She and her husband are looking for suggestions about further rehabilitation that would make managing him easier and that might facilitate increased independent functioning on his part. He is presently on no medications (she described him as "hypersensitive" to medications).

[Six years since his initial brain damage], the patient displays a clinical picture of neurobehavioral disturbances that makes it very unlikely that he could function independently or hold any type of employment. Despite apparent progress in many areas and intact skills (such as verbal communication), his distractibility, severe short-term memory loss, perseveration, and disinhibition (e.g., inappropriate touching) unfortunately result in a very poor prognosis for any significant increase in his ability to care for himself, to develop a meaningful relationship with another woman, or to work (at this far post onset of his condition). The increased touching behavior and apparent failure to recognize the emotional significance of objects he is touching (i.e., people) are in some ways suggestive of a human Klüver-Bucy Syndrome sometimes seen after significant anoxic brain damage.

My recommendations are that he receive more extensive in-home care and attention to alleviate the burden on his aging parents as well as to attend more directly to his problematic behaviors (i.e., touching). The individuals working with him need to be trained in behaviorally-based management of patients and/or should receive consultations from specialists in neurobehavioral disturbances. Due to the geographic location of their home, very little is available in the way of such services to the patient and his parents. An alternative approach would be to admit him to a residential neurobehavioral treatment program (which often runs for several months) and is often geared to patients with traumatic brain injury ...

I asked the neuropsychologist to send me pertinent literature relevant to Klüver-Bucy Syndrome. Gary had been evaluated dozens of times. Nobody had ever mentioned — nor had I ever heard of — Klüver-Bucy Syndrome.

I did receive the literature from Dr. B. An article from the *Journal of Neurology, Neurosurgery and Psychiatry* described bizarre behavioral disturbances in patients occurring during incomplete recovery from herpes simplex encephalitis. Aspects of their behavior were similar to descriptions of Klüver-Bucy in monkeys following bilateral temporal lobectomy.

The literature described four cases. In the first case the patient tended to pick up objects indiscriminately, ate everything within reach including feces and his urinary catheter, and drank large volumes of any liquid available including shampoo. In the second case, the patient would sit chewing paper, blankets and other objects, ate his feces, and would bite at pencils, fingers and other objects placed near his face. The third case involved a patient that attempted to eat a variety of objects early on during her recovery and eighteen months after the illness would still eat any sort of food placed in front of her. In the forth case, the patient walked around the ward picking things up at random, would often put them into his mouth, ate voraciously and drank liquids indiscriminately. Apparently, none of these patients demonstrated obviously abnormal sexual behavior, although one did tend to kiss or blow kisses to staff and other patients.

After reading the literature, I was confused; none of these symptoms related to Gary. He does not like to eat or chew non-food or inedible objects such as feces or blankets. He does love to drink, but not shampoo or urine — mostly Pepsi. He does touch people, sometimes inappropriately. He is disinhibited and unaware of his behavioral impact on others, but Klüver-Bucy?

As we drove home from Chicago, I felt disappointed, dissatisfied, and disgruntled. We put Gary through another series of evaluations at one of the best rehabilitation institutes in the country. Still, the prognosis, the recommended therapy, and where to go for it seemed — at least to me — muddled, unclear, and even more undefined than before.

The lawsuit was settled. We had the means to secure treatment for Gary, but where do we go for it? Nobody seemed to have concrete answers.

Of course, part of the problem is that we did not live in an urban area. I ran up humongous phone bills calling other facilities in the South, the West, and the Midwest. I collected a file full of literature from each one. A staff member at one recommended facility told me, "We can work with the behaviors for one month at a cost of $30,000, then we can make a decision if continued treatment is in order."

I scrutinized in excess of 30 facilities. Finally, I made an appointment with a rehabilitation facility in Milwaukee, one that had been in existence for many years.

Again, I forwarded all the medical records and engaged in repeated conversations with the neuropsychologist, who had also come highly recommended. We focused on a possible day treatment program. I explained that we would be willing to move to Milwaukee on a temporary, trial basis.

The day of the initial appointment we toured the facility. It seemed like a wonderful facility. My hopes began to escalate. *Have we finally found a suitable program for Gary?*

During the meeting with the neuropsychologist, Gary persisted with his usual perseverative questions — "How old are you? What year is this?" etc. After three or four questions, the neuropsychologist looked at him. "I'm not here to discuss my age or your age," he said. "Unless you have intelligent questions, I won't answer them."

I winced at his abrasiveness. Gary, puzzled and intimidated by this treatment, got up, looked visibly upset, then began to shake, and attempted to leave. My husband escorted Gary out of the room while I remained behind with the neuropsychologist. On the way out Gary — exhibiting his now heightened state of agitation — repeatedly asked, in a loud voice, for confirmation of his age: "FORTY-TWO — THAT'S

RIGHT?"

After they left, the room became silent. I sat there with my private thoughts: *I hope he has some answers for us; I would even consider moving to Milwaukee if necessary, living out of a motel, whatever it takes.* The neuropsychologist broke the silence.

"Gary shows signs of Tourette's Syndrome," he said. He noted that Gary's perseverative behavior becomes more pronounced and intense when he feels threatened and uncomfortable. "I don't think moving to Milwaukee and entering our day program is the answer," he said. "The move would be disruptive for Gary and might cause regression."

Desperate, I asked him to make recommendations for a facility able to work primarily with behavioral issues. He mentioned one in Wisconsin, but noted that there had recently been a changeover in personnel at that facility. "You could try that," he said. Then he gave me the name of a mother from Illinois who, like myself, had been through the gamut. "Why don't you call her?" he urged. "Her son's situation is similar. She might be able to give you some ideas about where she took her son for treatment. I know that, in the past, she was aggressively seeking out facilities."

I sat there somewhat stunned, thinking: *That's it? Check with another mother?*

Next, Gary had an appointment with a physician. The physician who had reviewed all of Gary's records in advance was out sick, so his supervisor agreed to see Gary.

We explained that Gary's speech had deteriorated — it was more accelerated and less comprehensible. Incontinence was also a developing problem. The supervising physician's report includes the following excerpts:

> Major complaints and concerns are deterioration in functional condition as evidenced by major problems in behavior. These include frequent poking, pinching, and perseverations as well as touching in an inappropriate manner. He also has limited cognitive and memory skills. With cues he is able to do some two-step memory tasks. Attention is extremely limited. He also has been noted to

have major deterioration in the above functions in the last two years. Coincidentally, after he tried a course of Prozac he has had incontinence of urine, but not on a consistent basis. Incontinence occurs usually at night, but he may be free from incontinence for several days at a time. There is no report of bowel incontinence. Currently he lives with his parents and they are coping as best as possible, and have adapted to some of the behavioral issues. A trial of Prozac, Haldol and various other medications in the past led to no successful resolution of the problems. The use of Haldol led to dyskinesia and therefore was discontinued. The parents in general are apprehensive about pharmacologic management of the problems.

.... it is felt that supervised inpatient brain injury rehabilitation is appropriate. This must be a significantly behaviorally oriented approach and may involve pharmacological management of the problem of behavior, attention span and memory dysfunctions. Prior to this, consideration may be given for a neurosurgical consultation, primarily to determine if hydrocephalus is significant enough through testing, which may include a CAT scan, MRI scan, etc. If it is indicated, consideration may be given for surgical intervention including shunt placement. A home-based behavioral management program is also suggested in order for the parents to handle him more appropriately.

In conclusion, Mr. Abrahamson has major residual problems resulting from the cerebral anoxia and the more recent deterioration over the past two years in terms of behavior. His parents were advised to make appropriate contacts for the above recommended approaches of care. At this time I am recommending discharge from [this facility].

Although inpatient brain injury rehabilitation was appropriate, taking Gary out of his environment and moving him to Milwaukee was not recommended.

The new evaluations in Chicago and Milwaukee led to a rash of new labels and new ideas: Klüver-Bucy Syndrome, Tourette's Syndrome, hydrocephalus; try L-Dopa, call another mother, check out another facility. With this most recent round of disappointments, I began to think that our search for the right treatment and the right facility was a mythical search for a pot of gold at the end of the rainbow — something elusive, maybe even fictitious.   Perhaps what we were doing at home — learning from trial and error, providing love and security — *was* the best treatment available for Gary.

I did get a neurologist to evaluate a new CAT scan to rule out anything structural — such as enlarged ventricles or hydrocephalus — that may be responsible for Gary's incontinence, speech deficits, and behavioral deterioration. According to the neurologist, the CAT scan showed "a little bit" of atrophy but no real change since his last CAT scan. He reported that Gary's condition was "very stable."

A few months later, we made arrangements to spend a month in Florida. We were somewhat reluctant to do so, remembering that Gary did not adjust well to our stay in Marquette while I was in school there. But after reading Dr. Laurence Miller's book, *Psychotherapy of the Brain-Injured Patient*, I decided to take the chance. I made advanced arrangements for Gary to see Dr. Miller, who lives in Boca Raton, Florida.

It turned out that Gary had a wonderful month in Florida. He adjusted exceedingly well to innumerable changes in his daily routine. Although there was some minimal poking behavior, our visits with Dr. Miller were quite productive. I attribute Gary's relaxed behavior in Dr. Miller's office to three factors: Dr. Miller himself was non-threatening to Gary; instead of the typical clinical motif, Dr. Miller furnished his office to look and feel more like a sitting room in a home; finally, my husband and I sat in on all sessions, which added to Gary's comfort level.

Dr. Miller made the following observations, among others:

> During the course of my sessions with Gary, he appeared to become somewhat more responsive to conversation, and more tolerant of less-than-total undivided attention. As expected, he does better in more familiar, structured situations. He was able to participate in many "Florida fun" activities with his parents during their stay here. On my recommendation, he purchased a book of cognitive games, and was able to attempt a number of them. There were

several setbacks, e.g., some aides couldn't handle Gary and quit, and he had an episode of poking behavior in a shopping mall. These setbacks probably represent a decompensatory response to the unfamiliarity of the new environment and new routine, as well as a tendency to become overwhelmed by overstimulation and complexity. The poking and hand-squeezing behaviors themselves seemed to be particularly resistant to verbal or behavioral control strategies ... .

Gary Abrahamson is a 43-year-old, right-handed, white male who shows a moderate-severe organic brain syndrome secondary to sustained anoxic brain damage caused by cardiorespiratory arrest. The present behavioral pattern is probably a stable one ....

The patient's parents have done an unusually meticulous and comprehensive job of caring for Gary, and I think they recognize that they have pursued every possible option in terms of his recovery and rehabilitation. The task now, as I see it, is to get Gary into some manageable and predictable routine that will enable him to make the most of his preserved abilities and achieve some reasonable and realistic degree of independence and autonomy. Despite his sometimes objectionable behaviors, there is a definite likeable quality to Gary that comes across despite his impairment. This will no doubt be a plus in terms of his gradual resocialization into the community at large. To this end, every effort should be made to strike a balance between providing Gary with enough social stimulation, without causing him to become threatened or overwhelmed. In addition, I have discussed with the family the necessity of making trust and guardianship arrangements [to assure that Gary is provided for in their absence]. I have also discussed some other specific recommendations with the family, and they will keep in contact with me by phone or mail as needed, and may schedule another series of sessions when they return to Florida next year.

By return correspondence, I asked him why he had omitted from his report the strengths he had observed during Gary's course of treatment. For example, in our informal discussions, Dr. Miller had commented on Gary's still intact "islands of intelligence" and strategic abilities (e.g., winning half of the tic-tac-toe games they played together). He responded as follows:

> Thanks for the photos. Gary looks great. At least one 43-year-old is photogenic.
>
> In response to your comments, clinical reports tend to be lopsidedly biased in favor of the negative stuff. That's because clinicians tend to focus on things that need improvement. However, as noted in your letter, I agree that Gary shows some definite areas of strength, in addition to the ones I outlined in my report, and certainly these should be taken full advantage of. As we discussed, I always hope for patients "not to read the textbooks" and show gains in functioning far beyond the time limits established for statistically typical cases.
>
> ... Good luck finding a knowledgeable psychiatrist, because precious few understand the special needs of TBI patients. But if you locate someone in your area, let me know and I'll be happy to send him or her some pertinent material on the subject from recent medical literature (you'd think these doctors would read their own journals). However, in the right hands, psychopharmacological approaches can be very useful for some TBI-related behavioral problems.

As Dr. Miller states, clinicians tend to focus on the negatives — those areas that need fixing. But families and caregivers, who sometimes rely upon hope to sustain themselves, need to hear the positives too. My whole theory in working with Gary is to build on his strengths.

At the end of the month, we returned to Michigan. It didn't take us long to realize that our stay in Florida gave us all a psychological boost. We left the sunshine and warmth of Florida and returned to the cold, blustery, snow-filled environment of Northern Michigan. Some days Gary needed a wool scarf draped around his face, leaving only his eyes exposed, just to leave the house. In the temperate Florida climate, by contrast, we found ourselves leaving the house more often, enjoying outdoor activities, and exercising more. We discovered — perhaps not surprisingly — that the sunshine, exercise, and more vigorous lifestyle helped us to cope, both mentally and physically. We began to discuss the benefits of spending more time in Florida, which included greater access to therapy options and a vastly improved psychological outlook for us all. Soon thereafter, we made arrangements to spend part of every winter in Florida.

During our next stay in Florida, I contacted a neuropsychologist in Sarasota. She was originally from Michigan and had accumulated thirty years of experience in the brain injury field. After meeting with us and studying Gary's medical records, she concluded that Gary was not a candidate for therapy at her clinic. Since it had been more than seven years since Gary's initial brain injury, she suggested that taking Gary out of his home environment would only serve to agitate and disrupt Gary, with little hope of any beneficial gains. She commended us on the care we were providing Gary and encouraged us to do more of the same.

Before we left, however, she suggested that Gary may be suffering from Alzheimer's disease. I was, for a moment, taken aback. I asked, "What basis do you have for that?" She explained that it has been documented that, after a brain insult such as Gary's, the onset of Alzheimer's is more likely. While it may not be possible to clinically document Alzheimer's in Gary's case, she cited his slight imbalance as he walks, unclear speech, and urinary incontinence as suspect factors. We left the clinic discouraged by this new possibility.

The next week, we kept our appointment with a small sister clinic in Ft. Myers, where we were staying. The day was filled with more evaluations. The inexperience of the young therapist with whom we met soon became clear, however. I think he was more interested in learning from us than he was capable of helping. We didn't go back.

Next, we visited another physician in Ft. Myers, one that was experienced in brain injury and came highly recommended. She signed prescriptions for Gary to receive both speech and physical therapy at a local hospital. Unfortunately, Gary was not cooperative. The therapies lasted about one month before they had to be aborted.

The physician then suggested that Gary be evaluated by a local psychiatrist, who was experienced with brain injury. He recommended drug therapy to deal with Gary's perseverative behavior problems. Up to that point, we had been reluctant to try pharmacological intervention, primarily because of Gary's past adverse reaction to it. However, it was the only avenue that we had not taken recently, so we agreed to a trial run. The psychiatrist explained that the antidepressant drug he was recommending, Paxil, would take three or four weeks before significant results would be observed. The drug, he said, had proven helpful in dealing with obsessive-compulsive behaviors. We tried the drug for about six months, gradually increasing the dosage. Though there weren't any negative side-effects, we didn't observe any improvements either.

About the same time, Gary began seeing a neuropsychologist at the local hospital. He made several observations and summations:

> ... Gary has been through numerous neuropsychological evaluations and treatment programs through the years, and has met some success. Success has often depended upon the quality of the relationship with the particular physical, occupational, or other therapists involved. I have reviewed a number of neuropsychological test reports dating back to June 1988, roughly eight months post injury. The most recent report was by Dr. Laurence Miller from March 1994.
>
> A review of earlier neuropsychological test reports indicate a relatively stable performance across the various functional realms. Most significant difficulties appear to lie on tasks of executive function, memory, and attention/concentration. More recent neuropsychological reports have focused primarily on Gary's behavioral problems, which have persisted throughout his course of rehabilitation....
>
> Since his injury his parents have continued to stand by him, and, in fact, spend most of their waking hours supervising and caring for Gary in some capacity. Gary evidently demands much attention from them and it is difficult for them to hold a conversation without becoming caught up in answering Gary's repetitive questions, and providing him with the nearly constant attention he demands when he is

near them. Gary is able to occupy himself for lengthier periods, however. He enjoys sitting in his jeep, listening to Beetles' music, and occasionally watching TV for longer periods.

Behavioral problems involving perseverative questions (e.g., "What's my age?") and inappropriate interpersonal behaviors (e.g., poking, flicking, and grabbing and patting others) have worsened during the last three years, according to the mother and father....

Gary's parents have dealt with these behaviors in a variety of ways. They have told Gary, "It hurts me," and asked him not to do it. They have [purposely tried to stay out of his poking range]. They have also tried ignoring the behaviors, but indicate that he eventually wears them out... It therefore appears that Gary has been on an intermittent schedule of reinforcement for both the physical and verbal inappropriate behaviors.

More recently, Gary's mother indicated they have taken him to see Dr. S., who prescribed Paxil 10 mg.qd. As of the third meeting with Gary, the mother felt that perhaps some of his perseverative behaviors had diminished. There is great fluctuation in the frequency and intensity of the problem behaviors on a day-by-day basis, however. For example, Gary seems to intensify the behaviors when he becomes agitated or situations occur which deviate from his usual routine....

Physical therapy reported of nearly constant patting, pinching, and poking or punching during at least one session. Gary seemed to do much better, however, in his speech therapy sessions where he was separated from the therapist by a table. In both situations, one or the other of the parents was present, but not actively involved in the therapy....

The neuropsychologist had several suggestions for us. First, since Gary's antisocial and problem behavior tends to increase when he is agitated or anxious, he suggested buying some audio tapes designed to relax Gary. In addition, we were to place a ball or other soft object in Gary's hands so he would be less likely to use his hands to poke or flick at others. Though Gary prefers listening to the Beatles rather than relaxation tapes, the idea about the ball was helpful. When we are at the mall, for example, sometimes we will push him in his wheelchair along the right side (so he only has the wall to his right) and put a Nerf ball in his left hand. This does seem to cut down on his tendency to poke strangers.

Next, he proposed a regime of behavior modification. Specifically, we were to count up the number of times Gary exhibited antisocial or problem behavior during a twenty-minute period. For example, let's say that over a twenty-minute period Gary did the following: asked about his age sixteen times, asked about your age twelve times, said "you're full of shit" twice, patted someone on the behind twice, asked what year it was nine times, and poked you in the stomach seven times. That would give us a baseline rate of 48 problem behaviors over a twenty-minute period. Then we were to divide the 48 problem behaviors by twenty to give us as average baseline rate of 2.4 problem behaviors per minute.

We were told to specifically ignore problem behaviors or provide only a quick answer and then move on — unless it hurt physically. We were then to take the average baseline rate (2.4 per minute), subtract one (leaving 1.4), and reward Gary with a dollar bill every time he had an average of less than 1.4 problem behaviors during a one-minute period. When Gary performed successfully for ten consecutive minutes (i.e. had been rewarded with one dollar during each of the last ten minutes) we were then to take the old reward rate (of less than 1.4 negative behaviors per minute) and subtract one, leaving a new reward rate (of less than 0.4 negative behaviors per minute).

According to the neuropsychologist, we were to adhere to this at home on a "fairly tight schedule." This behavior modification regime is known as "differential reinforcement of low rates of responding" — DRL for short! When I explained the recommendations to my husband, he responded: "You've got to be kidding? DRL? What's that stand for? Doctor's Really Lost-it? Or how about the Spanish translation — Doctor's Really Loco."

Having taken several psychology courses as part of my social work curriculum, I *do* appreciate the efficacy of behavior modification tools. However, clinicians must understand what an overwhelming task it would be for caretakers — already inundated with myriad responsibilities — to implement this on a minute-by-minute, day-by-day basis. While we subscribe to positive reinforcement techniques as a general matter, implementing such a specific, intensive regime is a little bit unrealistic.

16

LOVE AND SECURITY

We must not, in trying to think about how we can make
a big difference, ignore the small daily differences
we can make which, over time, add up to big differences
that we often cannot foresee.
- Marian Wright Edelman

This country is blessed with thousands of bright, dedicated clinicians. But, alas, the yellow brick road is mythical — there is no wizard.

Brain injury, it seems, is one of the last great frontiers of medical science; in a relative sense, it's undiscovered and undomesticated territory, a sort of badlands of the American West, unpredictable, full of wild animals and unknown dangers, a place where only fools rush in and angels dare to go. By contrast, there is seemingly no limit to what a family can do for a loved one with a brain injury.

Sometimes it's the little things that give comfort. The basic things, the day-to-day routines, the love, the security, the caring, the understanding, the patience — all of this, I have found — is more important to Gary's well-being than any drug or therapy program.

When Gary first came to live with us, even simple, normally enjoyable events such as eating were difficult. Between Gary's persistent perseverative questions, his desire for our full attention, unsuccessful attempts to carry on a normal conversation, and my efforts to encourage Gary to take bites of food, chew them, and swallow them, every meal became an unhappy event. I began to have swallowing problems and my husband experienced burning sensations in his esophagus.

Fortunately, we found a way to make mealtimes more pleasant for all of us. Now, my husband and I eat dinner early, while Gary is still on his afternoon outing with his aide/companion. This allows us to meet our need for normal conversation. As a result, our health problems have disappeared. Gary, in turn, is happier because he has all of our attention while he is eating (he is still egocentric), and I can focus on encouraging him to eat. We sit with him throughout the meal and virtually cater to him. He loves it!

Gary needs structure. We have learned that an hour's rest after dinner, before his evening outing, is beneficial to all of us. We shut our bedroom door, read the evening paper, and Gary, content, lies quietly until the hour is over. There's evidence, too, that Gary knows his routine and benefits greatly from structure. After dinner, he retreats to his bedroom on his own.

He used to wander through the house, asking perseverative questions all morning long. Now, I might bring him out on the patio, give him a Pepsi, and put on his earphones to listen to a Beatles tape. I look out the window, see a serene look on his face, and watch him tapping his foot and singing along.

My husband engages Gary in silly humor. They sing jingles from old commercials of 1960's and 1970's vintage. Gary Senior uses the Gillette Blue Blade jingle ("Look sharp, feel sharp, be sharp!") to cue Gary to shave every day. At other times, they may do the *Dragnet* sounds, Roy Rogers' "Back in the Saddle Again," or "Happy Trails to You." As they laugh and sing lyrics together, it really does my heart good to see this communication between father and son.

Even when Gary makes a remark like, "You used to spank me with a belt," my husband uses humor, responding, "Now I use hugs and kisses." We've all learned simple techniques that improve the quality of our life together.

Gary has a slight residual delayed swallowing problem. He has choked on a few occasions, requiring the Heimlich Maneuver. We must be cautious when selecting meals and usually have to cut his food pieces very small, much as you would for a young child. We must keep him focused while eating. Inattention, talking, or perseveration can exacerbate his eating problems.

He is generally more attentive and eats better when he really likes the food. So I make him all the things he liked as a kid — grilled cheese sandwich, spaghetti, steak, fried egg sandwich, pizza, cheeseburgers, and chocolate milk. When we celebrate his birthday, we wear hats, wrap presents, and I bake him chocolate cake. Many of these dietary items are not healthy, I know. But Gary doesn't have much in his life that makes him happy, and food is one of them.

During the early evening, we often go for a ride. Gary grew up in Escanaba so he often points out landmarks that were once important in his life. "The old A&W use to be right over there," he often says. To engage Gary in conversation, we usually set him up; for example, we tell him what a great hockey player he was (and he'll make some hockey conversation) or we tell him what a good worker he was (and he'll talk about some of the jobs he's held).

During the evening, we often watch television together. Gary used to poke, pinch, and become very obnoxious during this time. He didn't like competing with the TV for our attention. We addressed this situation by placing a huge pillow between Gary and us, making us hard to reach. Although there is still some perseverative questioning, Gary has adapted well to the routine we have established, and his attention span has increased: he actually watches and comments on segments of programs and commercials.

However, due to his memory and concentration deficits, Gary is unable to enjoy television or reading for long periods of time. But, if there are pictures or television material that is sexually explicit or suggestive, this is apparently more compelling, and Gary's interest and attention span increase.

When Gary first came to live with us, he would occasionally fondle himself. Initially, my husband forbid this behavior and tried to discourage Gary from engaging in it at all. Later, realizing that this was simply a manifestation of his normal sexual needs and desires, we would tell him to retreat into his room to engage in such behavior in private. Gary is not able to masturbate to completion. Apparently, he is unable to create or maintain the mental fantasy needed to complete the act.

Yet, the memory of sex and marriage is still etched in Gary's mind as a part of his pre-trauma life. Suddenly, through trauma, Gary was thrust into a dysfunctional sex life. Although Gary attempted to carry on a normal sex life after his brain injury, it was virtually impossible. Because of his memory impairment, he didn't remember having intercourse, and within a half-hour, would want to engage in it again. Apparently, he could perform, but he was egocentric — only interested in his gratification.

I was unaware of some of Gary's most inappropriate sexual behavior until I read them in the deposition Kris gave for the lawsuit. She recalled incidents where, in public, Gary would take out his penis, grab Kris by the legs, or take his pants down. Kris said these incidents would happen anywhere — on the street or in a restaurant, and often in front of their children. She stated that it was very difficult for her sons to see their father exhibit inappropriate sexual behavior, especially as they got older. She said the boys were exposed to a lot of things that she wishes they had not seen. Even now Gary sometimes asks where Kris is because, he says, "I want to make love to her."

One clinician even suggested a humane approach might be to "solicit a prostitute" for Gary to provide an outlet for his desires. Although I didn't dismiss it out of hand, I did consider it bizarre: *A mother seeking sexual release for her son?* I was raised in an era when most parents hardly even discussed sexual topics with their children; it was hushed up, swept under the rug.

Since we live in a small, rural area and since AIDS is a reality, I do not intend to follow through on this — humane as it may seem to some. I am just too uncomfortable with it. Still, having worked so hard to meet his other needs, I wonder if I would feel differently if we lived permanently in a city with sex therapists and other options. Gary doesn't live in a vacuum. His pain is real; I see it daily. He has very human needs for fulfillment, just as we all have.

We try to make sure that Gary spends a few hours almost every day — either with us or with his aide — in the community. He walks, exercises, enjoys picnics in the park, walks in the mall, picks strawberries, plays basketball, pool, ping pong, fooz ball, and air hockey. He also likes to play the slot machine at a nearby casino. He is fascinated by numbers and money, excited just to have a pocketful of nickels. He has gone dancing, goes to restaurants for pizza and burgers (his two favorite foods), attends band concerts and sporting events.

I continually search out and introduce new activities. A few years ago, I even experimented with guitar lessons. Gary surprised us all. Despite his short-term memory deficits, he was able to learn several chords. He did become frustrated, however, and we had to abort the lessons. Gary needed something more gratifying — something with immediate results. The lessons might take months, years before he could actually strum a tune. However, he's receptive to instruction, willing to try anything. Presently, I'm looking for a good art teacher to work with him. This might prove to be his niche, given his tremendous pre-morbid creative aptitude.

One of Gary's previous aides was convinced that he could safely drive an automobile. She worked with him almost every day. Before long, Gary was proudly driving, never requiring any verbal assistance. He is a cautious, considerate driver fully aware of his responsibilities as he drives through the streets of our town in heavy traffic areas. Though at the time Gary's driving was a novelty, and we enjoyed observing his new-found freedom, we take a more prudent approach today; driving with a brain injury could put others at risk and result in significant legal liabilities.

I have also introduced Gary to computer therapy. This is a controversial area. Some clinicians have concluded that it does not improve memory. Others disagree. While the jury is still out on whether computer therapy is an effective means for rehabilitating memory, I have used it to enhance Gary's preserved memory. Potentially, it has the capability to improve Gary's spatial relationships (geography software), calculation abilities (math software), and overall vocabulary and spelling. From experience, I've learned that cognitive activities are more productive in the morning. In a clinical setting, you fill the slot they have available; if that spot is 3:00 p.m., when Gary's blood sugar level is low, so be it. At home, I am in control.

Recently, we took him to a couple of concerts — Kenny Rogers and Tom Jones. Gary started to cry when he heard certain songs that apparently had sentimental value to him. The only other time I have seen his eyes well up with tears is in church. I don't know what it is — perhaps a moving sermon, perhaps other families remind him of his own nuclear family, or perhaps church somehow inspires a greater realization of his condition — but sometimes his eyes tear up. Usually, however, church is the one social activity that seems to transform Gary, a lost soul, into a person free from the abyss of his amnesia. He takes communion and tries to sing the songs. Sometimes, he seemingly experiences an inner peace, one that shuts out the ugly vice of confusion that normally grips him.

While in Florida, we took Gary to a major league baseball game. We planned it so we were able to see Mitch Webster, who at the time played for the L.A. Dodgers. Mitch, who attended Gary's church in Kansas, had prayed with us at the hospital while Gary was still in a coma. He never knew Gary's outcome. It was so heartwarming to see his warm response to Gary. Before the game, he escorted us behind the locked gates at the ballpark where we took pictures of him and Gary together. Gary remembered him, and later, sat through the whole game yelling, "Hey, Mitch!" every time Mitch came onto the field. Gary joined the crowd in yelling "Hey, Strawberry!" and "Da-a-a-rrell!" The crowd was in a heckling mood and Gary fit right in.

We also take Gary out to eat occasionally. These outings, however, can be stressful. Sometimes he becomes loud or disruptive and we have to leave before our meal is done. Though I can't always prevent this disruptive behavior, I do have some control over how he looks and presents himself. I make sure that he has nice things to wear, has brushed and flossed his teeth, combed his hair, shaved, and put on cologne. People in the community often comment on how exceptionally well-groomed he is. After all, if he is going to command attention, at least he will look good while he is doing it!

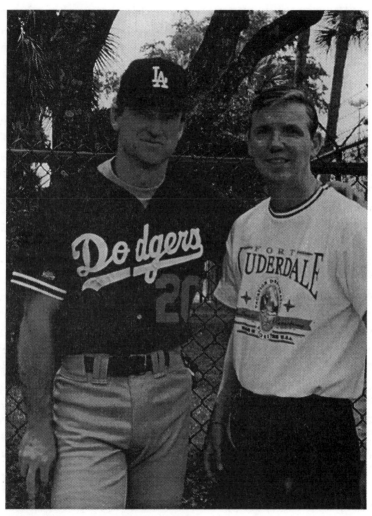

Gary with friend Mitch Webster, 1994.

But there are risks associated with mainstreaming Gary into the community. For example, during hunting season one year Gary was in a fast food place with an aide. He went into the bathroom while she waited. Suddenly, she heard screaming and yelling. She went into the men's bathroom to find Gary on the floor and a hunter from Detroit kicking him.

"What's going on?" she screamed hysterically. "He has a brain injury!"

This insensitive man, a former police officer from Detroit, showed no emotion or remorse. He explained that he thought Gary was a homosexual because of his touching and poking behavior. Gary's body was black and blue the next day.

Another day, an aide had Gary order his own Pepsi at the food court in the mall. Gary ambled to the counter.

"What's your age?" he asked.

The clerk didn't answer, so Gary asked again.

"Women don't tell their age," she retorted. "And it isn't polite to ask."

Perhaps feeling insulted, Gary became more insistent and loud. His aide apparently stood by, silent.

Then, "Get him away from me!" the clerk screamed. "Get him away from me!"

A competent aide could have averted that acceleration with some redirection. Gary is unaware of his behavioral impact on others, and he is troubled by perceived slights or situations such as I described, not fully understanding why he was treated so rudely. He holds the thought for hours. Fortunately, these incidents are isolated. Most people in our community know of Gary and his disability, and make special efforts to speak to him and make him feel comfortable.

Then again, sometimes it's the aide that we have to watch out for. One week, Gary had a few black and blue marks. At first, we attributed it to a bump in the shower or something like that. When they increased, we began to suspect the aide. We thought that maybe she had a low tolerance level for Gary's remarks or poking behavior and took countermeasures against him. We confronted her about it. She denied it, then quit the following week. Lo and behold, the marks cleared up. I had no idea that people would do such a thing. With this experience behind us, we now periodically inspect Gary's body for any suspicious marks.

Gary's tendency to poke, pat, and pinch people — apparently an attempt to get someone's attention or a reaction — wasn't present until about four years ago. At the time, Gary had a male aide who, in retrospect, may have caused undue harm. He was indifferent and insensitive. He left Gary unattended in his car for extended periods. He even lost Gary once and had to call the police to help locate him. My first recollection of Gary's poking behavior began about this time. His stomach was huge, and Gary insisted on poking it, or pinching him. Gary apparently sensed this man's indifference to him, and Gary poked and pinched him to get his attention, acknowledgment, and respect.

Sadly, Gary's poking and pinching behavior became perseverative — his now standard way of getting attention when ignored, or even when he is not ignored. The search for a behavioralist who can treat this perseverative behavior is never ending. But even if one target behavior is successfully treated, that is not the end of the story. We have found that one perseverative behavior may subside, and another one appears or becomes more intense. It's almost like a water hose with several holes in it; you can put your fingers over a couple of the seepages to slow them, only to observe other leaks become more intense.

We must take special care in orienting people that work with Gary. Many don't realize how difficult he can be and initially conclude that Gary's idiosyncrasies "won't bother me." Then, when they show up for the first time, and Gary greets them with a how-come-you're-so-fat-and-ugly question, they get a better idea of the challenge they are about to confront. We have to tell them that they haven't been singled out: "He says that to everyone." It's true. He claims even skinny people are too fat.

But Gary can be unmerciful. Trying to teach Gary good social graces, I insisted that he come say good-bye to one particular aide. Gary came to the door and said, "Good bye, Wilma, I hope I never see you again."

Most often, he is not aware of having said anything cruel. If one of us reminded him, he would emphatically deny he could say something like that. Another aide he greeted for the first time was taken aback when Gary blurted, "Wow, you have big breasts." Not knowing what to say, she responded: "Yes, I've been told that before."

Although Gary is disinhibited — says just about anything that comes into his head — he does not confabulate as he did before. In earlier years, to hide his inability to remember facts, Gary would invent explanations, create a world to replace what was lost or forgotten. Fortunately, he no longer has a need to do this. I tell him, "You've come a long way, baby, and the journey is not over yet!"

A few years ago, Gary attended his 25th high school class reunion. This was the second class reunion he attended since the brain injury. He went to his 20th class reunion with Kris. At the earlier reunion, Gary lacked attention span, was frustrated, and left before the social hour ended. My guess is that the experience actually caused some painful awareness of how different he is from his peers.

The more recent reunion went well. Apparently, it was more gratifying not only because Gary had made some improvement, but also because his classmates are more aware of and sensitive to his plight.

At my request, the following remarks were read by one of his classmates at his 25th reunion:

> Fellow classmates:
>
> In October of 1987, almost six years ago, Gary Abrahamson suffered sudden death while jogging. Subsequently he was revived and as a result, he has a brain injury. At the time of the tragedy, Gary was doing his clinicals to become a nurse/anesthetist.
>
> After struggling through a coma, Gary has had to relearn basic skills in order to walk, talk, and swallow. He's come a long way on the road to recovery and continues to make slow progress.
>
> He does not have day-to-day memory but he does remember school and classmates. For that reason, he has expressed a strong desire to be present this evening — to renew old friendships and be a part of the life he loved and remembers.
>
> Gary has brought with him a memory book and asks

that his fellow classmates sign it, to help him have a memory of being here tonight.

Let's ask Gary to stand up so we can welcome him and show him we care.

Gary attended both the Friday night mixer and the formal Saturday evening dinner/dance. Carmella, his aide at the time, is a sensitive friend and beautiful person. She escorted him, calling herself Gary's "date." Her reports were glowing. Apparently, Gary beamed when he was recognized before the class. And, when his name was called for a door prize, he went up to the stage to collect it on his own. He delighted in the attentiveness of his peers.

We — my husband and I — basked in the good news that Gary was able to attend a social function in its entirety and actually enjoy it.

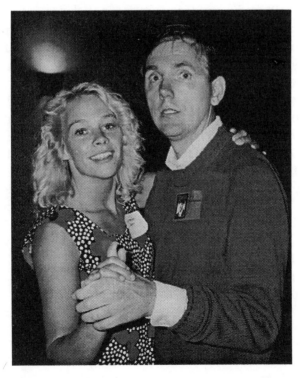

Gary and Carmella share a dance at his 25-year high school reunion, 1993.

As Carmella continued to tell me about the evening, a moment of sadness brought tears to my eyes. "Gary is an excellent dancer," she exclaimed. "We both cried as he reminisced with music from the 60's." She went on: "He put his head on my shoulder and with soft sobs, spoke of how he missed his wife and longed for his life before — how it used to be!"

Carmella was one of Gary's best aides and we were sad to see her move on. Over the years, however, I've become proficient at hiring aides and know what to look for. We have found that sensitivity and a caring, sincere attitude is far more important than educational credentials.

After the night of his reunion, Gary seemed relaxed but a bit tired. As parents, it did our hearts good to hear that Gary, overall, had a good evening. When it was time to go to bed, I took him to his room and helped him into his pajamas. He looked around and seemed content, surrounded by memorabilia of familiar faces and sentimental items. In his room, there is a picture of Mitch Webster, his friend, a member of his Kansas church, and professional baseball player. On the wall is a poster of Gordy Howe, his favorite hockey player; his brother Jeff got the poster signed by Gordy Howe at a reception in Washington, D.C. and gave it to Gary for Christmas. Also on the wall are a couple of photographs of Kansas landscapes, which Gary took while pursuing his photographic interests. On the dresser is a picture of the Beatles (one of his favorite groups) and a trophy Gary won for coming in second place in a 10k run in Kansas. And on top of his pillow rests a stuffed poodle — reminders of the two dogs Gary's family owned, Chantilly Lace and Pepper.

I put him in bed, pulled the covers over him, patted his face, and told him I love him.

"You sure are handsome," I said.

"I know," he replied.

17

COMIC RELIEF

A laughing man is stronger than a suffering man.
                                    - Gustave Flaubert

Humor is highly valued. It is, for most of us, an important part of our lives. It can be used in so many ways — to put
people at ease, to consolidate relationships, to communicate
more effectively, and to provide comic relief during an otherwise stressful situation. In fact, laughing is known to release
endorphins, the same brain-secreted chemicals responsible
for "runners high," the euphoric feeling some people experience after a long jog.

Norman Cousins, former editor of the *Saturday Review*
who was diagnosed with a painful, degenerative spinal disease, used laughter to cope. He reasoned that if negative
emotion was bad for health, its opposite might have a beneficial effect. Cousins watched multiple episodes of Candid Camera and Marx Brothers movies because he found that ten minutes of belly laughter gave him two hours of pain-free sleep.

In his 1979 book, *Anatomy of an Illness*, Cousins tells of
the fun he had with a particular nurse while in the hospital.
He called her the *we* nurse, because she irritated him by asking everything in terms of *we* — such as "how are *we* today?"
or "have *we* filled up our urine specimen cup?" One morning,
he filled his urine specimen cup with apple juice. When the
we nurse saw it, she said, "My, *we* are a little cloudy today."
He took it back and said, "Yep, better run it through again,"
and drank it. "The look of shock on her face," he said, "was
priceless."

Before succumbing in 1991 to a brain tumor, Republican

strategist Lee Atwater reportedly read Cousin's book and spent some of his final nights watching *The Three Stooges* and other humorous video tapes.

Some say laughing — at least the hearty belly laughter type — is a form of internal jogging. Your face warms, blood pressure increases, and heart rate goes up. Recent research suggests that humor may have a direct effect on the body's ability to fight infection. Apparently laughter boosts the body's production of "killer" white blood cells. Deepak Chopra, the well-known lecturer, says there is proof that the tears of laughter contain a completely different group of minerals than tears of grief. Today, some hospitals even offer "Humor Rooms" stocked with tapes, games and toys.

One developmental psychologist, aware of the medicinal affect of laughter, deals with rush-hour traffic jams by wearing a giant elephant nose. Traffic barely moving, he straps on the nose and waits for a reaction. Soon people are staring and laughing.

While the Abrahamson family has always had a good sense of humor, it has — perhaps by necessity — been taken to new heights (or lows) in the course of Gary's brain injury. Some of the humor is characterized by a level of crudeness that would not likely have survived or even been tolerated in the pre-brain injury Abrahamson family. Today, however, there is a wild-west-anything-goes-locker-room-whatever-works-let-it-all-hang-out attitude toward humor of which, I dare say, even radio shock jock Howard Stern would be proud. And for that I don't apologize; it helps us get through the day.

Oftentimes, the humor serves a very functional purpose. You see, Gary doesn't always have regular bowel movements, and a few years ago he ended up with a bowel impaction for which he had to undergo a rather uncomfortable procedure. Today, we look for subtle warnings (for example, Gary will bend over slightly) that signal a need to have a bowel movement. Gary Senior uses humor — together with appropriate incentives — to ensure that Gary does his bodily duty. One day, I overheard the following exchange between Gary and his dad:

Dad: Gary, do you have to go to the bathroom?

Gary: How do you know I have to take a shit?

Dad: Well, you're leaning forward. And besides, I'm your dad — it's my job to know such things.

Gary: Oh, you're full of shit, aren't you?

Dad: Come on, Gary (taking him by the arm).

Gary: Where are we going?

Dad: We're going to the bathroom.

Gary: Why do I have to listen to you?

Dad: Because I'm the boss.

Gary: The boss of what?

Dad: The boss of the shit house.

Gary: What's your age boss?

Dad: Sixty-five big ones.

Gary: You're the boss of the shit house — that's right?

Dad: Yep. Let's go. I'll give you $5 for each turd.

Gary: (laughter) That's right? You'll pay me to take a shit?

Dad: Yes sir. Five bucks a piece.

After several minutes in the bathroom, Gary appears in the living room.

Gary: You owe me $15 bucks, boss.

Dad: Wait. I have to see the evidence.

Gary: I already flushed them.

Dad: OK. I'm leaving to do some errands, but I'll cash a check and give you the $15 when I return.

Two hours go by. Meanwhile, Gary's short-term memory problem has erased the debt from his mind. Gary's dad arrives home.

Dad: Gary, here's your $15.

Gary: What's this for?

Dad: You made three turds at five bucks a piece. A deal is a deal.

Gary: You mean you pay me to take a shit — by the turd?

Dad: That was the deal.

Gary: (laughter) You're crazy, Dad. Had I known you

were going to pay me, I would have shit my brains out. (laughter)

Early on, shortly after Gary's brain injury while still in the hospital, he screamed at me to leave.

"Get on a plane and go home!" he wailed.

I was weeping when the nurse came to intervene.

"Larry," the nurse said (she got his name wrong), "you shouldn't treat your mother like that!"

Gary turned to me. "What did Larry do to you?" he asked. "If I get a hold of Larry, I'll kill him!"

Occasionally, Gary becomes constipated, and we usually treat it naturally — with prune juice. One time, we apparently gave him too much prune juice because his constipation soon gave way to diarrhea. That resulted in an accident, one that required immediate attention. Gary, Gary Senior and I — we all took a rather awkward position as we commenced cleaning Gary up. When Gary began to shift and move, I blurted: "Wait, wait, there's shit all over." Confused, laying on his side, Gary cocked his head toward me, and — eyes wide with a serious demeanor — said, "*WHO* shit in my pants?" While it now seems like strange and demented humor, the absurdity of the situation prompted Gary Senior and I to laugh hysterically — as if we'd been exposed to toxic levels of Jim Carey. Even Gary drew a smile. That brief interlude didn't move us any closer to getting Gary cleaned up, but for a fleeting moment, it seemed to lighten the load.

Gary's comment, as funny as it was, helps reveal something about his brain injured personality. Gary may have asked "who shit in my pants" because he really was confused about who *did* do it. Or he may have asked the question as part of a weak attempt to mislead us, and help preserve his dignity — a form of denial: As if to say, "Who did that because I certainly didn't do it."

Throughout the day, we also monitor Gary for signs that he needs to urinate. Again, the signs are subtle; sometimes he gets slightly agitated or begins to shift weight from one foot to the other as if to perform a warning dance.

At that point, we usually inquire: "Gary do you need to go to the bathroom?"

Typically — even though he clearly needs to go — he retorts: "No, do you?"

By then he is usually unable to hold the urge for more than a few minutes, so we have to act quickly. However, if a toilet is not easily accessible — for example, if we are driving in the car — time may run out, and we have to clean him up and change him.

Sometimes, however, he'll simply give us no warning at all. Sitting on the couch or in the car, he may simply announce: "I'm taking a piss right now." Then, when I try to change him, I'll say, "Gary, take off your shorts." He'll say, "No, you take off your shorts."

Other times, he would simply urinate, then live with it — generally without awareness or complaint — until we were able to sniff out the problem and address it.

Then when he does make it to the bathroom, I praise him. He'll say, "What's the big deal about taking a piss?"

Gary has a scar running from the top of his chest to the top of his belly as a result of heart bypass surgery. Changing his shirt, looking at his scar in the mirror, he turned to his dad and said:

"Who cut my chest open, Dad?"

"The doctor," his dad responded.

"If I ever get hold of him, I'll kick his ass," Gary retorted.

"But, Gary, the doctor helped you — the doctor from Green Bay," he said.

(silence) "You know the doctor from Green Bay, right Gary?"

"No ... it's bad enough knowing you," Gary retorted.

Later that day, his dad wanted to see if Gary remembered the comment about kicking the doctor's ass.

"Hey Goose," his dad said (an affectionate name for Gary).

"I'm not Goose," he said, "I'm Gary Abrahamson, Jr."

"I think I'm going to go kick his ass now," his dad declared.

"Kick whose ass?" Gary queried.

"My own," his dad said, not wanting to bring up the reference to the doctor.

"Need any help?" Gary asked.

Recently, we visited Gary's local doctor.

"Hi Doc," Gary said. "How old are you?"

"He's fifty-one," I said, not wanting the doctor to feel compelled to reveal his actual age.

"I'll take that!" the doctor said.

Gary looked at the doctor, studied him, then blurted, "Oh, you're full of shit, aren't you Doc?"

"Well, yes — I've been told that before."

"But I bet you've never been told that by a patient — especially at the *beginning* of an appointment," I said.

"That's true," the doctor said, "but it helps keep you humble."

During lunch one day, Gary wasn't eating his sandwich. Trying to use humor to get Gary to eat, his dad said, "C'mon Gary, you have to eat your sandwich or we'll throw it out." Gary's response: "No, we'll throw you out!"

Although Gary's witticisms may — at least to the uninitiated — suggest hostility toward his dad, we know not to take these comments seriously. In fact, when Gary's dad isn't around for a while, Gary will ask, "Where is the old bastard? I miss him."

Occasionally, our other children — Jeff or Vicki — will call the house while Gary Senior and I are either outside or downstairs (where we can't always hear the phone). If Gary is nearby, he will answer it. One time, Jeff called with some news that he wanted to pass on to his father. Gary Senior and I were outside in the yard, and Gary answered the phone.

Gary: Hello.
Jeff: Hello Gary.
Gary: Jeff?
Jeff: Yes.
Gary: You're my brother?
Jeff: Yes.

Gary: How old are you?
Jeff: Thirty seven.
Gary: How old am I?
Jeff: Forty five.
Click. Gary hangs up.

Jeff calls back.
Gary: Hello.
Jeff: Gary, why did you hang up on me?
Gary: I don't know. What's your age?
Jeff: Thirty seven. Is Dad there?
Gary: Yes.
Jeff: Can I talk to him?
Gary: Why?
Jeff: Because I have something important to tell him.
Gary: Why?
Jeff: Because...
Gary interrupts: What's my age?
Jeff: Forty five.
Click. Gary hangs up.

Jeff waits ten minutes, then calls back.
Gary: Jeff?
Jeff: How did you know I'd be calling back?
Gary: What's your age?
Jeff: Thirty seven.
Gary: It's 1996 — that's right?
Jeff: That's right. Gary, could you go get...
Click. Gary hangs up.

One day I told Gary that I "will give you 20 bucks if, for the next five minutes, you can refrain from asking your age or what year it is."

"Holy cow," he said, "twenty bucks — that's right?"

"That's correct," I said. *10 seconds later:*

"What's my age?"

Most summer evenings, we take Gary for a ride down by the beautiful lake front in Escanaba. He loves to relax in the back seat, legs crossed, chewing a piece of gum. He watches people feeding pigeons in the park, kids playing on the massive public jungle gym called the Castle, young adults playing volleyball, basketball, and tennis, and families laying on blankets, enjoying snacks and each other's company, and listening to band concerts. On the way back home, we sometimes stop to get a yogurt cone.

As we were making our way across town, Gary sat up, back arched, and said:

"Stop," he said. "I want to get out."

"Why do you want to get out?" I said.

"I want to get out and go there," he responded.

"Go where, Gary?"

"Go there," pointing at the town's only adult book store. "I want to get out and go to the dirty book store."

After a couple of seconds of silence, checking each other for a reaction, we all laughed, including Gary, who apparently realized the absurdity of stopping at such a venue *with his parents*.

Gary's brain injury has left him very disinhibited — the normal taboos, norms of polite behavior, and fear of embarrassment are not present. Gary will say just about anything that comes into his head. Recently after watching a television commercial about a particular feminine product, Gary turned to me and asked, "Mom, do you have a yeast infection?"

On another occasion, Gary came out of the shower and said:

"Man, look how big I am," pulling at his genitalia like a rubber band. "Dad, do you have this much hair down there?"

"C'mon, Gary let's towel off," said his dad, trying to change the subject.

"Dad, why am I so big down there?" Gary insisted.

"You're just lucky I guess," said Gary Senior.

"No, I'm lost," said Gary.

Gary's comments make you want to laugh and cry at the same time.

One afternoon, Gary Senior, Gary Junior and I took a drive to the grocery store. They both waited in the car while I ducked inside to do some shopping. Later that evening, Gary

Senior revealed part of the conversation I had missed.

Gary Senior (jokingly): Gary, what are you going to get me for Valentine's Day this year?

Gary: How about a good kick in the ass? (laughter)

Gary Senior: Come on Gary — isn't that what you got me last year? Can't you think of something better to get me this year?

Gary: Yes. How about two kicks in the ass?

One morning at the breakfast table, Gary was speaking in a loud tone — as he tends to do sometimes, perhaps without total awareness as to how loud he is. So I asked him: "Gary, why are you so loud?"

"Because I'm nuts," he responded.

"Why are you nuts?" I queried.

"You'd be nuts too if you lived with you and Dad as long as I have!"

Gary is acutely aware of his environment — down to the most minute aspect. He is the first to notice an ant on the floor, a dirty spot on a mirror or wall, or a speck of dirt on someone's shoe. One morning Gary turned to his dad during breakfast and said, "Why is that crumb under your chair? What are you — a pig?"

He is also acutely aware of people's looks and focuses in on certain, usually negative features. Gary has become increasingly critical of people's looks — even his own. Perhaps this is a function of his memory being stuck in 1979. Of course, we all looked younger back then. Looking in the mirror, scrutinizing his hair which is slightly graying at the temples, he exclaims, "Why am I so old?" A few hours later, he turns to me and says, "You looked much better before. Why is your hair so short now? I liked it long."

Gary tells it like it is. You may be talking to him, and he'll blurt: "You have bad breath." Or "Why is your butt so big now?" Or "How come your teeth are so yellow." Wherever we take him — restaurants, malls or anywhere else, he comments on how fat people are, how yellow their teeth are, or how ugly they are. Sometimes his perceptions are correct, sometimes not. Gary makes these derogatory comments so often, his dad has made a game of it. It goes something like this:

Dad: All right Gary, let's play word association. I say a word — you finish the phrase. All the phrases will describe me. Ready?
Gary: Ready.
Dad: Bad...
Gary: Breath.
Dad: Yellow...
Gary: teeth.
Dad: No...
Gary: Hair.
Dad: Big...
Gary: Nose.
Dad: Who does that describe?
Gary: You. (laughter)

Recently, the three of us — Gary, Gary Senior, and I — were watching television. Gary was sitting at a slight angle to the television, inspecting his father and I. After a few minutes, Gary asked: "Why are you both so fat and ugly now?"

"Gary, you shouldn't make those kinds of statements — it makes people feel bad," I said.

"I'm sorry, Mom — I didn't mean that," he said. "You're beautiful — well, you're just a little bit homely with those glasses on."

Then, a few minutes later: "Dad, why are you so fat and ugly?"

"Gary, that's not a very nice comment."

"I'm sorry, Dad." Then: "Dad, why are you so fat and beautiful?"

"Just for that comment, I'm going to kick your ass," his dad says jokingly.

Not to be outdone, Gary responds: "Ya, I'll sit on your face and fart in your eye."

Several months ago, we were traveling together on a plane. Traveling with Gary on *any* type of public transportation is *always* risky. I managed to get a seat in the front row of our section so Gary wouldn't be able to poke or pester anyone seated in front of us. We tried to keep him occupied for the two-hour trip. Toward the end, he became restless. When he began to get loud, his dad tried to counsel him. Then all of the sudden, in a loud, clear voice: "Dad, why did you used to spank me with a belt?" When he did not get an answer that satisfied him, he got up, stood in front of his dad, faced the entire passenger section, and shouted: "Why did you spank me with a belt?" During the final 15 minutes of the flight, Gary had everyone's attention. We laugh about it now.

In the mornings, I sometimes help Gary brush his teeth, comb his hair, and dress him. Once in a while, he'll glance down at my chest, look me in the eye, and exclaim, "Ma, why do you have such big breasts?" Then, "Let me see how big they are." I try to ignore these comments or redirect him to another subject. But before I am able to, he'll usually get one last comment in: "They're monsters!" Meanwhile, Gary Senior is in the living room having a good belly laugh.

Some psychologists might criticize our reaction to Gary's inappropriate behavior. They might claim that we are helping to perpetuate this behavior by finding humor in it. But, then, the psychologist doesn't have to live with Gary, endure his insults, or change his urine-soaked underwear. To the critics, including those in the ivory towers, I find at least a partial defense in the words of Theodore Roosevelt.

> It is not the critic who counts, not the man who points out how the strong man stumbled, or where the doer of deeds could have done better. The credit belongs to the man who is actually in the arena, whose face is marred by dust and sweat and blood, who strives valiantly, who errs and comes short again and again, who knows the great enthusiasms, the great devotions, and spends himself in a worthy cause, who at best knows achievement and who at the worst if he fails at least fails while daring greatly so that his place shall never be with those cold and timid souls who know neither victory nor defeat.

We realize that much of this is dark humor, if it is humor at all. Yet, laughing helps us all cope. In fact about the only time the *old* Gary peaks through the *new* Gary is when he is smiling, laughing, and cackling. Despite his brain injury, he is really quite witty.

Preschoolers laugh on average 400 times a day. The average adult laughs only 15 times daily. Perhaps we really can learn from our kids!

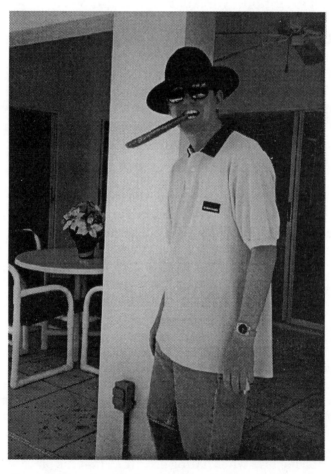

Gary cracks a cigar-filled smile during a lighter moment.

18

REFLECTIONS

We begin to live when we have conceived life as a tragedy.
                                                              - W. B. Yeats

As we march steadily ahead through life, one foot over the other, continuing our uphill climb, it is worthwhile to gaze over our shoulders, down the path we have just taken, and reflect; viewing the vista from a higher point on the hill, we gain new perspectives, learn from past deeds, and, hopefully, ease the burden of our climb.

Adjusting to our new lifestyle with Gary — one of accommodation, acclimation, and assimilation needed to assume the 24-hour care of an adult with a brain injury — was difficult. For my husband, the transition was agonizing; he continued to talk of a placement for Gary long after I had resolved that he would never be institutionalized. Both my husband and I yearned for our former life, one with no real problems, one that now seems — at least by comparison — self-indulgent, unstructured, and carefree.

Before the tragedy, we lived in a self-manufactured cocoon. We thought that tragedy doesn't happen to people like us — only to others. We were comfortable with our life: dining out, dancing, trips to wherever. Our kids were raised, and we had earned the right to revel a bit — or so it seemed.

Then, in an instant, without warning, tragedy struck; we were consumed — first with his survival, then his rehabilitation, then his destiny. It became clear that Gary's recovery may take a long time, or may never come. I felt guilt and disgrace knowing that my son was not normal. It took some getting used to. Then, there came a defining moment — Gary came to live with us and his ultimate welfare depended on us.

Committing ourselves to take care of Gary every day, every month, every year, possibly for the rest of our lives was prodigious. Though he is our son, the decision did not come without reservations. It is hard enough to deal with having an adult son who has a brain injury; it required an even higher calling to commit the rest of our lives — our so-called golden years — to caring for him.

But time was on Gary's side. With time, we broke out of our cocoon; with time, we were able to accept what happened to Gary; with time, we became less self-centered and more sensitive to the problems and hurts of others; with time, we came to accept our new role in caring for Gary. Today, my husband is comfortable and happy with his role. Time and a sense of resolution have brought inner peace to us all. Time and new perspectives on life has made us better people than we were before the tragedy. Now, I sometimes question what kind of a person I used to be — perhaps not anyone I would admire!

Now, our greatest concern is Gary's welfare after we are gone. He won't have the kisses, hugs, encouragement, and the kind of unconditional love that only his parents can provide him. But, we are doing everything we can to make sure that, in the long-term, Gary's monetary and physical needs are looked after.

As I look back, we experienced some very dark days. The first few years after Gary came to live with us were the most difficult. During those days, turmoil, struggle, and uncertainty pervaded our lives. Inner peace seemed little more than a distant dream.

My initial reaction, my way of coping, was to pour myself into Gary, to run myself ragged, and nearly run my husband out of the house. My life bordered on a self-imposed martyrdom. I was angry when well-meaning clinicians advised me to get a life or to take time out for myself. I didn't heed those warnings. I didn't trust anyone else with Gary. I was totally devoted to him and wasn't, frankly, able to derive pleasure from anything else. I soon learned that this form of martyrdom nearly doomed us. I learned the hard way that you need to come up for air. In the long run, caregivers who balance duty with occasional respite stay stronger, think more clearly, and are better equipped to handle the immensity of their role.

Another way I coped was through education. I needed to understand this foreign new world that was controlling our lives, that had propelled us into a future we could not imagine. I filled my head with information. I sought information from hospital pamphlets, journal articles, relevant books, the Brain Injury Association, and conferences. I sought information from course work in my degree program. Each bit of information gave me a deeper understanding of what was happening to Gary — and to us. The dogged pursuit of information, enlightenment, and answers was productive; this process of discovery also proved to be a great coping mechanism.

My initial expectations for Gary's recovery were very high. I hoped, unrealistically, that we could — somehow, eventually — bring about a near-complete recovery. I was naive to the pernicious character of brain injury. Over time, my expectations became more realistic. I eventually came to grips with the fact that Gary will never be the person he was before.

With the advantage of hindsight, I now realize that those unrealistic expectations helped to motivate me. The hope that Gary would recover was an increased inducement to care for him, to advocate for him, to go the extra mile.

Think of a mother that is able to muster the adrenaline-packed strength to lift a car that is pinning her young child. Would she have even attempted such a feat if she didn't have somewhat unrealistic expectations? What if she had concluded that she has absolutely no chance, no hope, no realistic expectation that she could lift a 3,000-pound vehicle? Hope — slim though it may be — provides the incentive to attempt it. To be sure, there were days when our hope was just to survive the next minute, the next hour, the next day. But we always had hope. Without it, there is despair. Never, ever lose hope.

Hope increased my determination. Determination gave me strength. I found out how important it is to advocate, to be tenacious. I never accepted a "no" from any agency — at least not on the first go-around. I talked to supervisors, called department heads, called the state offices, called and wrote my representatives in Congress. Most of the time, success was achieved only after I went well beyond that first "no."

Our religious faith also gave us the strength to carry on in the face of great difficulty. Praying in the hospital chapel for Gary's survival, I experienced a tingling right down to my fingertips — a sensation unlike anything I had ever experienced before.

Even when Gary lay in a coma undergoing seizures, even when I was told he would only live a couple of weeks, my faith didn't waver. Our prayers *were* answered — Gary survived. Even the neurologist concluded that a higher power must have intervened.

Months later, I prayed for complete healing. And when it didn't happen on my timetable, I became angry with God. Regretfully, I fell away from the church. I wondered how a loving God could leave Gary in this state — permanently lost in time and space, a hell on earth.

Now I have come to accept this fate for Gary and ourselves. I believe we are better people for having been touched by this tragedy. I feel close to God again. Gary has joined our church. He attends both Sunday mass and a weekly healing service regularly. Now, ironically, he says *he* prays for *us*!

Gary's tragedy transformed all of us. I can't say that life will ever be the same, but I can say, finally, that I am at peace. One mother of a disabled child once described the feeling:

> It's as if you were planning a trip to Italy and your mind was filled with images of the Vatican, gondoliers, and wonderful meals of tomato-laden pastas. And then you find, suddenly, with little warning, that you're going to Germany. Germany is a fine place; there are lots of nice things to do and see and eat there. . . but it isn't Italy. You feel disappointed, but eventually you learn that Germany is a fine place to be, with charms of its own.

To a disinterested observer, Gary's problems might appear unresolved. This is particularly true if resolution means restoring Gary to his pre-trauma self. However, resolution also means to persevere, persist, see it through, hang tough, fight, and never — no never — say die. This attitude can spell success in any endeavor; this attitude has brought solutions that work for us.

Unending love of our child and a sense of responsibility to him has helped us see it through. Not everyone could or would do it. And there were times when I didn't think we could do it. But we've done it, and I wouldn't want it any other way. Commenting on his mother's suicide, well-known lawyer Gerry Spence suggested that no one escapes this world without some trauma or tragedy, and it's from these experiences that we grow — not from the joyful times.

To be sure, I grieve for and miss the *old Gary*. There are times when I see a certain smile, hear a particular laugh, detect a gesture reminiscent of the *old Gary*, and tears flow spontaneously.

But I also love the *new Gary*, and I can truthfully say that our lives would be empty without him. With him, we are a family again — perhaps a slightly dysfunctional and unconventional family, but a family nonetheless. He has transformed *carefree* parents into *more caring* parents. He has given new meaning to our life, a reason to start each day, to stay strong and healthy. This acceptance, this transformation, this resolution didn't happen overnight. It has taken years. Time is a masterful healer.

I find comfort in the Serenity Prayer.

God, grant me:
-the Serenity to accept the things I cannot change,
-the Courage to change the things I can, and
-the Wisdom to know the difference.

19

FUTURE HOPE

A decent provision for the disabled is the true test of civilization.
- Samuel Johnson

Our children are our future. Yet, traumatic brain injury is now America's number one killer and cause of disability among young people, age 15-24. Motor vehicle accidents, sporting accidents, falls, and increasing violence are some of the major causes.

Two million people a year suffer brain injuries, many of which lead to irreversible and debilitating loss of function. Even the fortunate ones require years of rehabilitation, medical follow-up, and integrated community services. The cost in dollars, including medical treatment, rehabilitation, and disability payments is — even by conservative estimates — a staggering $25 billion yearly. The cost in terms of human suffering is immeasurable. But this is an epidemic that, normally, *is not* covered in the newspapers, seen on television, or treated in the movies. No, this is a silent epidemic. It quietly claims its victims without the sort of public alarm that would accompany any infectious disease outbreak of this magnitude.

In fact, a few decades ago, Gary may have simply died as a result of his heart attack. Medical technology was able to bring him back to life. Today, a decade after his cardiac arrest, we have ever enhanced capabilities to respond to life-threatening situations. During that medically-critical "golden" hour after an injury, highly trained personnel are able to air-lift victims to state-of-the-art trauma centers and administer miraculous lifesaving procedures. As a result, thousands of our sons and daughters, brothers and sisters, fathers and mothers have survived a brain injury and must now be cared for.

Despite the prevalence of brain injuries in this country, a coordinated, focused health care program aimed at traumatic brain injury (TBI) prevention and treatment does not yet exist. Such is not the case, for example, with cancer, heart disease, and many other maladies. Unfortunately, many health and social service agencies overlook, exclude, or inadequately service TBI survivors. Many rehabilitation programs are designed for people with a physical disability, not a cognitive disability. Moreover, there is inadequate research on techniques to repair damaged brain cells, improve memory loss, and improve cognitive functions.

Congress recognized these shortcomings in 1988 when it recommended that the Secretary of Health and Human Services (HHS) establish an Interagency Head Injury Task Force to identify gaps in research, training, and medical management. In 1989, the interagency task force recommended development of a national strategy to address prevention, acute

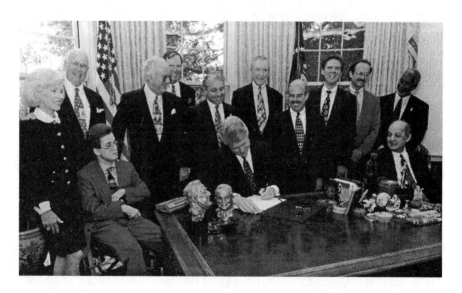

President Clinton signs the TBI Act into law. (L-R) Puddin Foil, Philip Foil, Martin Foil, Rep. William Hefner (D-NC), George Zitnay, PhD, Rep. James Greenwood (R-PA), President Clinton, Sen. Orrin Hatch (R-UT), Rep. Henry Waxman (D-CA), Rep. Frank Pallone (D-NJ), Dr. Harold Varmus, Dr. David Sacher and James Brady.

and long-term care, and community reintegration of TBI survivors.

In July 1996, following several failed attempts to pass federal legislation to implement these recommendations, the U.S. Congress cleared and the President signed into law legislation (H.R. 248, P.L. 104-166) which does the following:

Prevention. In order to reduce the incidence of brain injury, it authorizes the Centers for Disease Control (CDC) to provide grants or carry out projects to identify effective strategies for the prevention of TBI, including public information and education programs.

Diagnosis and Treatment Research. In order to better treat traumatic brain injury, it authorizes the National Institutes of Health (NIH) to award grants or contracts to support basic and applied research to develop new methods for effective diagnosis, measurement, and post-injury monitoring of brain injuries; to develop and evaluate therapies that retard, prevent, or reverse brain damage; to develop programs that increase the participation of academic centers of excellence in brain injury treatment and rehabilitation research and training.

Improved Access To Services. In order to address gaps in public services for brain injury victims and their families, it authorizes matching grants to states for demonstration projects aimed at improving access to health and other services. To qualify for the grants, the states are required to establish a State Advisory Board — composed of representatives of public agencies and private groups involved in brain injury as well as brain injury survivors and the families of brain injury survivors — that will hold public hearings and make recommendations to the State on ways to improve brain injury services coordination. By July 1998, the Secretary of HHS must submit a report to Congress describing the findings and results of the demonstration projects and programs.

Brain Injury Study. It authorizes the Secretary of HHS, working through the Public Heath Service agencies, to conduct a study to determine the incidence and prevalence of TBI; to identify common therapeutic interventions which are used for the rehabilitation of individuals with such injuries; to analyze the effectiveness of rehabilitation interventions; and to develop practice guidelines for the rehabilitation of traumatic brain injury.

National Conference. It authorizes NIH to conduct a national consensus conference on managing TBI and related rehabilitation concerns.

Definition of Traumatic Brain Injury. For purposes of this law, it defines traumatic brain injury as an acquired injury to the brain. It does not include brain dysfunction caused by congenital or degenerative disorders, nor birth trauma; however, it may include brain injuries caused by anoxia due to near drowning. Importantly, it gives the Secretary of HHS the authority to revise the definition as necessary.

This law, without doubt, will lead to greater understanding of the causes of TBI and ways to prevent it. The development of practice guidelines and standards of care should result in better, more consistent outcomes. The research activities could help identify early intervention strategies to help optimize medical and rehabilitation outcomes, minimize costs, and decrease the lengths of stay after acute injury; research could also help identify the best environments to address long-term recovery needs of people with severe physical, cognitive, and behavioral problems following TBI as well as the best methods for educational, psychosocial, and vocational reentry into the community for people with TBI.

The state demonstration projects will lead, hopefully, to increased coordination of medical, rehabilitative, and social services at both the federal and state level. Over time, public and private institutions will develop more appropriate and accessible treatment programs and facilities.

The study will give us authoritative statistics on the number of TBI cases as well as the extent of injuries, which will sensitize state and federal legislators to the prevalence of TBI, and may lead to further publicly-funded improvements in the

TBI health care system and human services bureaucracy.

While it may take several years before the real benefits of this legislation are realized, current and future victims of brain injuries should applaud its passage. Special recognition should go to the national Brain Injury Association for its diligent efforts to shine appropriate light on the need for reforms. And congratulations should be given, among others, to Senators Orrin Hatch (R-UT) and Edward Kennedy (D-MA), Representatives Jim Greenwood (R-PA) and Frank Pallone (D-NJ) as well as former Representative Jim Slattery (D-KS) for their legislative support.

Finally, a heartfelt thank you goes to James Brady, President Reagan's press secretary who was brain injured in the 1981 assasination attempt, for his willingness to personally promote the passage of this legislation.

What You Can Do

Passage of this legislation is not the end, however; it is just a new, hopeful beginning.

First, this legislation (Public Law 104-166) simply *authorizes* the above-described grants, studies, and consensus conference. This is a three-year authorization which will expire in July 1999. During each of these three years, Congress must take separate actions to *appropriate* monies for these authorized programs. Unless Congress provides funding in an appropriations bill for the authorized programs and activities, the legislation will do little or nothing to help current and future brain injury victims and their families.

Second, the legislation's definition of traumatic brain injury (TBI) is too narrow. The definition arbitrarily excludes those who suffer an acquired brain injury as a result of losing oxygen during a heart attack or a stroke. However, to their credit, the legislators recognized that this definition may be too narrow and so provided the Secretary of Health and Human Services explicit authority to revise the definition as necessary.

To address these two issues, write a letter to your U.S. Congressman and both of your U.S. Senators. On the next page is a sample letter. If you don't know the name of your

U.S. Representative, you may call (202) 225-3121. If you don't know the names of your U.S. Senators, you may call (202) 224-3121. Since these numbers are often busy, you may want to simply call the local number for your Congressman or Senator to get from that office all of the names and addresses that you need. Since you are a constituent, they will be happy to provide you with that information.

Date
Your Name
Your Address

Representative _____:
U.S. House of Representatives
Washington, D.C. 20515
-or-
Senator _____:
U.S. Senate
Washington, D.C. 20510

Each year, two million Americans suffer brain injuries, many of which lead to irreversible and debilitating loss of function (costing society a staggering $25 billion annually). During the 104th Congress, the House passed under suspension of the rules, the Senate adopted by voice vote, and the President signed into law long-needed, bi-partisan and non-controversial legislation (H.R. 243, the Traumatic Brain Injury Act, now Public Law 104-166) to expand efforts to reduce the incidence of brain injury, identify new treatment methods, and improve access to and coordination of services for the brain injured and their families. This was a three-year authorization; it still needs to be funded each year through the appropriations process.

Also, this public law defines "traumatic brain injury" as follows: "an acquired injury to the brain. Such term does not include brain dysfunction caused by congenital or degenerative disorders, nor birth trauma, but may include brain injuries caused by anoxia (oxygen deprivation) due to near drowning. The Secretary (of HHS) may revise the definition" as necessary. This definition is too narrow and arbitrarily excludes those who suffer an acquired brain injury as a result of losing oxygen during a heart attack or a stroke. By giving explicit authority to the Secretary of HHS to revise the definition, the legislators recognized that this definition may be too narrow.

Therefore, I am writing to request that you do the following two things:

1) Make sure that the Traumatic Brain Injury Act (P.L. 104-106) is fully funded for this and the next fiscal year. Talk to your colleagues on the Appropriations Committee if necessary. If this Act is not funded each of the three years for which it is authorized, its purposes will not be accomplished.

2) Write a letter to the Secretary of Health and Human Services (HHS) in order to let the Secretary know that the definition of traumatic brain injury is too narrow and request that the Secretary use the authority P.L. 104-106 gives to expand the definition of traumatic brain injury to include those that acquire a brain injury as a result of losing oxygen during a heart attack or a stroke.

Please write to let me know what action you have taken on these two requests. Thank you.

Sincerely,

Your Name

Then, to give full effect to the legislation in your specific state, your state government must take certain actions in order to get the matching federal funds authorized under P.L. 104-106. Therefore, you may also want to write your *state* elected officials. On the next page is a sample letter.

Date
Your Name
Your Address

State Representative (or Delegate) _____:
State House of Representatives (or Delegates)
          -or-
State Senator _____:
State Senate
          -or-
Governor _____:

Each year, two million Americans suffer brain injuries, many of which lead to irreversible and debilitating loss of function (costing society a staggering $25 billion annually). During July 1996, the U.S. Congress cleared and the President signed into law long-needed, bi-partisan and noncontroversial legislation (H.R. 243, the Traumatic Brain Injury Act, now Public Law 104-166) to expand efforts to reduce the incidence of brain injury, identify new treatment methods, and improve access to and coordination of services for the brain injured and their families.

To make this federal legislation work, however, each state has to take action of its own. For example, this federal law provides for matching grants ($2 of federal money for each $1 of state money) to states for demonstration projects aimed at improving access to health and other services for brain injury victims. However, in order for our State to qualify for these federal matching grants, our State must agree to establish a State Advisory Board — composed of representatives of appropriate public agencies and private groups involved in brain injury as well as brain injury survivors and the families of brain injury survivors — that will hold public hearings and make recommendations on ways to improve brain injury services coordination. Application for these grants must be made to the U.S. Secretary of Health and Human Services.

Therefore, I am writing you to request that you take appropriate action to assure that such an Advisory Board will be established in our State and that our State applies for and receives federal matching grants to help fund the activities of this Board.

Please write to let me know what action you have taken on this request. Thank you.

Sincerely,

Your Name

If you are a brain injury victim or a family member of a brain injury victim and have information or recommendations that could be helpful to an Advisory Board that has formed in your state, you may want to write the Advisory Board or ask if you may testify before it. If you need further information about brain injury, available services, or further advice on how to become actively involved in helping to address this epidemic, call or write the Brain Injury Association as well as your state brain injury organization.

Right now, no cure exists for brain injury; therefore, there must be a continual focus on preventing traumatic brain injuries in the first place.

Although a brain injury can happen to anyone, the typical victims are young people — especially young males whose behavior often puts them at risk. In this age of fast bikes, roller blades, skates, skate boards and snow boards, we must see to it that our children's heads are protected — not only for the sake of potential victims but for society at large, who ultimately foots the bill in terms of health care costs and loss of productive citizens.

The brain is the most fragile of human organs. Knees, elbows, wrists, legs and arms usually heal fine. The brain has a very poor ability to heal itself. We can't stop accidents altogether, but we can reduce the incidence of brain injuries caused by them through greater use of helmets. Helmet use can be increased by a combination of legislative and educational approaches.

If you need further information about brain injury, available services or further advice on how to become actively involved in helping to address this epidemic, call or write the Brain Injury Association, as well as your state brain injury association, listed in Appendix B.

Ultimately, one of the most important things we can do is to increase the awareness of this epidemic among our state and federal legislators. Concerned citizens in New York State have taken an innovative approach using the artistic talents of its brain injury population. Despite their injuries, it seems that many victims of TBI have wonderful artistic talents. One Colorado man, who reportedly became a well-paid sculptor after his brain injury, claims an accidental blow to his head left him with heightened artistic talents. Every year, the Brain Injury Association of New York puts together an art exhibition in the North Concourse at the Empire State Plaza. This exhibit, which gets press coverage, offers a chance for New York's brain injured population to communicate their experiences on canvas before thousands of state workers, legislators, lobbyists and other members of the public — a public that remains largely uninformed about brain injury and its manifestations. In an era where hundreds of groups are trying to bend the ears of legislators, innovative approaches such as this can be effective.

Perhaps one day we'll see the development of a nationwide art exhibition held simultaneously in Washington D.C. and in every state capital. It will be called TBI-Art-Across America. And it will raise the awareness of brain injury to a higher level. And it will lead to the passage of new laws. And future victims of brain injury will be a well-recognized, distinct population among health care providers and public assistance professionals. And persons with brain injury will never be at risk of "falling through the cracks." And, finally, there will be no need to write books like this.

Appendix A

FAMILY MEMBER STATEMENTS

Man is the only animal that laughs and weeps;
for he is the only animal that is struck by the difference between
what things are and what they might have been.
- William Hazlitt

Statement from Gary Senior, Gary's Father

The phone call informing us about Gary's apparent cardiac arrest left me stunned and in shock — then a dreaded message: "Gary isn't expected to live through the night." I remember crying and at the same time trying to comfort my wife. It is still painful to conjure up the thoughts and feelings of the nightmare that followed.

Gary did survive the night, and in the days to come, he survived crisis after crisis. I had to take one day at a time. He was in God's hands and how I prayed that my son would live! Those months were chaotic and painful.

As time passed, I became ambivalent. One moment, I was grateful that he was spared — the next moment, angry at losing the "old Gary." At times I questioned God, asking *Why?*

I was saddened that Gary had lost his wife, his family, and his ability to work or care for himself. Every day, when he laments about his losses, I feel the pain again.

When Gary came to live with us, there were times when I felt overwhelmed with the awesome responsibility. Like many father-son relationships, ours had been bittersweet. We weren't always close; we didn't always agree.

Gary's tragedy has transformed me. I'm a better human being and a better father — more sensitive, more caring, and in some ways, more like a "mother." In retrospect, it seems to me that God gives all of us a reserve tank to run on, but most people are not challenged to draw on that reserve tank. I think perhaps God was preparing me long ago through my involvement with sports; we get by through teamwork, doing what we have to do, sometimes challenging ourselves to do more than we thought we could.

I have watched my wife and her loving interactions with Gary. I have learned through her example. I understand now how all-consuming a mother's love is. Nothing on earth can compare with the unconditional love of a mother. This is the *true* meaning of love.

The grace of God gave me the strength to do my part. Inspired by my wife, I became a better father and caregiver.

Ironically, a heightened loving relationship was spawned from Gary's tragedy, an event that has affected me more deeply than anything else in my entire life.

I loved the "old Gary," but my love for the "new Gary" is deeper. I love him mentally, and show it physically in hugs and kisses every day. And he responds, "I love you, Dad. I've loved you from the day I was born."

I have a new job in retirement; it's far more meaningful, more fulfilling than the work I did to support our family during the children's growing-up years. I'm truly grateful to God for allowing me to love and care for Gary in my old age.

Yes, I still mourn my son's losses, and my losses as a result, but then I think of the alternative: no Gary at all, and I thank God for answering our prayers. The three of us are a family again.

Escanaba, MI

Statement from Vicki, Gary's Sister

The quality of my life has never quite recovered from that fateful day: October 25, 1987. The phone call I received that Sunday evening as I sat on the floor in my bedroom, I will never forget. When I picked up the phone and heard my mother's voice, I knew something was terribly wrong. She began to explain why she was calling me, and my mind jumped to the conclusion that my dad had a heart attack, but as I listened more closely, I realized she wasn't talking about my father; she was talking about my brother!

You always hear this kind of story from someone else, but the words being generated were coming from me: *My brother might not live to see tomorrow!*

As we made our plans to go to Gary's bedside in Kansas, we all thought we were in a terrible dream. We thought we would wake up to find everything back to normal; this was not happening to our family. If it was happening to our family, it was going to turn out okay. But everything did not turn out okay. We got more than we prayed for when we asked God to *just keep him alive, no matter what.* The Lord didn't give back the same Gary we had all those previous years, but returned my brother without his memory.

The effect on my life was probably more than I could really deal with at that time. I only know now just how devastated I really was. The trip to Kansas to say good-bye to Gary was so chaotic as we scrambled to get to his bedside, because he wasn't expected to live through the night. There were so many lows while we sat and prayed at the hospital waiting for Gary to come back to us.

At night, I shared Gary's bed with his wife Kris. One night, we were awakened by a phone call from the hospital telling Kris that she needed to come immediately and sign papers for an emergency procedure that needed to be performed. At this point, the emotional drain on my system had physically caught up with me and I became very ill. I could only literally crawl on my hands and knees out of bed and down the hall to be of assistance to Kris as she got ready to go to the hospital to meet this current crisis. From that time on, I had many physical afflictions due to the stress.

I returned home after one week, still in a state of shock, of course. My parents stayed in Kansas waiting for Gary to show signs of improvement. I drove to my home from Milwaukee, a distance of some 240 miles, in great despair. I returned to my life and work, but my mind was a thousand miles away. At that time, I held two jobs. My main job was for my father, running his dry cleaning business in my home town, and the other as a part-time waitress at a local supper club. I didn't know how badly I was affected by the anguish that was happening in my life until I tried to return to normal life at home and work. It was exhausting enough keeping my mind on task at the cleaners during the day. Then, during the evening, when I returned to my waitress position, I realized the severity of my condition. That first night I returned was like another page out of a bad dream. I couldn't keep my concentration even to take an order, let alone remember how and where to serve it. This was just before the holidays, notoriously the busiest time of year. I knew I wasn't up for this additional stress emotionally, so I gave notice that night that I would be taking a leave of absence.

Gary's episode was like a cancer inside of me; I was unable to contain the emotions I was feeling. Since Gary is only about fourteen months older than I, thoughts that I would be the next victim haunted me. I became very paranoid and intensely aware of my breathing pattern and heartbeat. The worst times came when I wasn't busy. I was convinced that 18 days after my 37th birthday was a possible D-Day for me, for this was the day when Gary's life began to stand still. One particular Sunday, sitting on my couch, I became tense. I put my fingers to my throat to count my heartbeats: *Are they too faint, too slow, or maybe they're too fast?*

My mind was obsessed with doom and gloom for my own future and health. I became very weak in every sense of the word: my voice was soft and it took too much energy for me to speak with any volume. When I attended church to pray for Gary on Sundays, I would ask the Lord to spare me, hoping that this would not happen to me, too. While in church I found that I couldn't sing in my normal voice, so I would mouth the words. But the worst times came when I was alone in my house. When the kids would leave for school, I would have what is called a panic attack. I was afraid to be away from the phone because I was sure I was going to need to call for help. I wrote down all the emergency numbers and would carry them from room to room while rushing to get out of the house so I could be around people that could help save me.

I missed being the independent person I used to be: strong, calm, and unruffled. I even feared driving out of the city limits alone in my car. As the weeks marched on and Gary's prognosis didn't change much, I felt the spirit of my life diminish, too.

Now that many years have passed, I still feel a piece of my spirit has never returned. My days are not as bright and my nights, not as peaceful. Still, a portion of the old Gary will always remain in my memories — I miss him so! Music serves as a catalyst, setting off a beacon in my heart when I hear his favorite artists on the radio. I think of his tall, trim, model-material physique, his classy approach and his confident manner. I am saddened when I think of the Gary we have with us now, the Gary with the frail shell, whose shoulder droops as he shuffles his feet to walk, asking the same questions over and over again: "What year is it? How old am I?" My love for Gary hasn't changed. Perhaps it has even grown stronger. As profound as our loss has been, he has suffered so much more — losing his very personality, his wife, his children, and the purposeful life he once lived. My only consolation in all of this is that Gary now resides with my parents and couldn't be more loved or better cared for. Gary is the recipient of a kindness so complex that even he, with all of his limitations, can recognize that this truly is the meaning of love.

West Bend, WI

Statement from Jeff, Gary's Brother

Two monumental things happened in October 1987: Black Monday's stock market crash and my brother's cardiac arrest which left him brain damaged. One event made the headlines of almost every newspaper in the nation; the other went largely unnoticed — except among those close to Gary. Politicians and financial practitioners still talk about that month. And so does Gary's family — but for a different reason.

I vaguely remember that late October evening in 1987, when I first learned of the event that would bring permanent and devastating change to Gary's life. I'd just taken a job in New York City, and my wife and I were settling into our new home. The last time I'd seen Gary, two years previous, he was in Washington, D.C. for my marriage — looking fit, trim, healthy, and, as one of my ushers, sporting a black tux.

As I watched him proudly escort my mom down the aisle that day, vignettes of my relationship with Gary began to emerge: *And he scores!* As kids, we used to roll up a sock, shut the hallway doors, and play hockey using, for sticks, the face of our hands or strategically bent hangers. He was Gary-Gordy Howe and I was Boom-Boom Jeffrion. I remember Green Bay Packer football games, golf outings, informal barbecues; I think of his fondness for nicknames, including those he had for me: "little bro," "the dude," and when I was much younger, "pee-cat" (let's just say my kidneys lacked a certain all-night capacity until I was about eight years old).

I don't recall who first informed me of Gary's cardiac arrest that fateful evening, but I do remember talking to Gary's doctor. He gave me a report on Gary's condition and said it would be appropriate for family members to come to Kansas. *Appropriate for the family to come?* In shock, I didn't draw him out but concluded that this was code language for "Get out here as soon as you can if you want to see your brother one last time before he dies."

Once in Kansas, despite negative reports from the doctors, we remained steadfastly hopeful. We talked, consoled, and prayed. For me, it was not my first time in Kansas. Four years earlier, I'd gone to Kansas to visit my brother and his family. Fresh out of undergraduate school, with no firm commitments, I stayed a year, working side by side with Gary at the same firm. Now, standing over him, watching the respirator plunge up and down, I thought how sadly ironic it was to remember that sunny morning in Kansas when Gary passed me near the finish line of the 10k race we had entered.

After a week in Kansas, I returned to New York to resume settling into a new home, a new job. The Kansas experience left me remarkably unsettled. I felt heart palpitations for weeks and became concerned about my own health. Looking out my 32nd floor Park Avenue office window, seeing the slow-moving traffic, hearing the faint but constant roar of horns, didn't help allay my fears. I worried it would take too long to get to a hospital if something happened; I fastened the emergency number to the back of our home phone; I made an appointment with a cardiologist for a full battery of tests. And thoughts of Gary and his condition continued to haunt me. I began to make frequent stops to pray and meditate at a church near my office.

Things are more stable now, and Gary survived — just as we had prayed. But he hasn't recovered. The brain injury has taken away the Gary we knew. Medical know-how was able to avert death. Yet it did not, and does not, have the capability to give him back his life. It's all so sad and tragic. Anyway, I love him and congratulate my parents for their determination to make the best of the situation. With my dad's imaginative and distinctly Norwegian humor and my mom's perseverance and nurturing spirit, I know he is, for the moment at least, as happy as possible given the circumstances. I also know it has been a hardship.

Washington, D.C.

Statement from Alexis, Gary's Aunt and Friend

A secretary in the department of a University I was attending gave me the message. My first thought was that Gary Senior had a heart attack. But I re-read the note and it said Gary Junior had a heart attack and to call Great Bend. I rushed home to tell Glenn and we immediately called to find that Gary was in the hospital, in critical condition, and not expected to live. Glenn and I prepared to go to Great Bend to see Gary perhaps for the last time. I remember on our way from Colorado to Kansas we saw a star fall from the sky and we both thought that perhaps Gary had died as we watched the star fall.

We arrived in Great Bend to find that Gary was still alive. We did get to see Gary and we wanted to help in any way we could. Glenn and I watched Gary's boys for several days. Some small things about that time stayed in my memory. I remember making oatmeal for Leif and helping Arlo with his homework. But mostly, I remember praying to God to spare Gary's life.

I had become close to Gary and his family through Glenn, Gary's uncle. Glenn and I had visited Gary almost every summer since 1978. In the two years prior to his cardiac arrest, I had developed an even better rapport with Gary because he was attending college and we talked about that. He had also become a more devout Christian and we talked about religion. It seemed even more of a tragedy that Gary had a cardiac arrest because he had gotten his life together. He had direction and a purpose. He had his family and he had God. It is hard to understand.

I still visit Gary every summer, but now it is very different. He no longer cooks up specialty meals for Glenn and me. In fact, Gary doesn't cook at all any more, and Glenn is no longer living. Gary does not play catch with his boys. His boys are in another town. Gary now spends his time with his parents. Thanks to his parents, Gary has the means to live a comfortable life. Since the time of his cardiac arrest when Gary lay in the hospital bed, he has improved so much. The doctors said he would be a vegetable if he survived. But Gary isn't a vegetable. He still looks handsome, appears healthy, and when he smiles, looks like the Gary I used to know. This summer when I visited, Gary dug into a banana cream pie his mother made. He had a huge smile and his face lit up. His blue eyes twinkled and he looked just like the Gary I used to know and visit. He always had a sweet tooth.

I commend Patt and Gary Senior for their care of Gary and their diligence in seeing that Gary has everything he needs. I still pray for Gary, and I miss him.

Muncie, IN

Appendix B

BRAIN INJURY ORGANIZATIONS

National Association

Brain Injury Association, Inc.
1776 Massachusetts Avenue, N.W.
Suite 100
Washington, D.C. 20036
(202) 296-6443
Family Help Line: (800) 444-6443

State Associations

Alabama Head Injury Foundation
(205) 328-3505
(800) 275-1233

Brain Injury Association of Arizona
(602) 952-2449
(800) 432-3465 (in state)

Brain Injury Association of Arkansas
(501) 771-5011
(800) 235-2443

Brain Injury Association of California
(916) 442-1710
(800) 457-CHIF (in state)

Brain Injury Association of Colorado
(303) 355-9969
(800) 955-2443 (in state)

Brain Injury Association of Connecticut
(860) 721-8111
(800) 278-8242

Brain Injury Association of Delaware
(302) 475-2286
(800) 411-0505

Brain Injury Association of Florida
(954) 786-2400
(800) 992-3442 (in state)

Brain Injury Association of Georgia
(404) 817-7577
(888) 334-2424

Brain Injury Association of Illinois
(708) 344-4646
(800) 699-6443 (in state)

Brain Injury Association of Indiana
(317) 356-7722
(800) 407-4246

Brain Injury Association of Iowa
(319) 291-3552
(800) 475-4442 (in state)

Brain Injury Association of Kansas and Greater Kansas City
(816) 842-8607
(800) 783-1356 (in state)

Brain Injury Association of Kentucky
(502) 899-7141
(800) 592-1117 (in state)

Brain Injury Association of Louisiana
(504) 775-2780

Brain Injury Association of Maine
(207) 626-0022
(800) 275-1233

Brain Injury Association of Maryland
(410) 448-2924
(800) 221-6443 (in state)

Massachusetts Brain Injury Association
(508) 795-0244
(800) 242-0030 (in state)

Brain Injury Association of Michigan
(810) 229-5880
(800) 772-4323 (in state)

Brain Injury Association of Minnesota
(612) 378-2742
(800) 669-6442

Brain Injury Association of Mississippi
(601) 981-1021
(800) 641-6442

Brain Injury Association of Missouri
(314) 426-4024
(800) 377-6442 (MO, KS and IL only)

Brain Injury Association of Montana
(406) 657-2077
(800) 241-6442

Brain Injury Association of Nebraska
(402) 761-2781
(800) 743-4781

New Hampshire Brain Injury Association
(603) 225-8400

Brain Injury Association of New Jersey
(908) 738-1002
(800) 669-4323

Brain Injury Association of New Mexico
(505) 889-8008
(800) 279-7480 (in state)

Brain Injury Association of New York State
(518) 459-7911
(800) 228-8201 (in state)

Brain Injury Association of North Carolina
(919) 833-9634
(800) 377-1464

Brain Injury Association of North Dakota
(701) 281-0527
(800) 279-6344 (in state)

Ohio Brain Injury Association
(614) 481-7100

Brain Injury Association of Oklahoma
(405) 635-2237
(800) 765-6809 (in state)

Brain Injury Association of Oregon
(503) 585-0855
(800) 544-5243 (in state)

Brain Injury Association of Rhode Island
(401) 725-2360

Brain Injury Association of South Carolina
(803) 533-1613
(800) 767-9701

Brain Injury Association of Tennessee
(615) 264-3052
(800) 480-6693
Brain Injury Association of Texas
(512) 467-6872
(800) 392-0040 (in state)
Brain Injury Association of Utah
(801) 484-2240
(800) 281-8442 (in state)
Brain Injury Association of Vermont
(802) 446-3017
Brain Injury Association of Virginia
(804) 355-5748
(800) 334-8443 (in state)
Brain Injury Association of Washington
(206) 451-0000
(800) 523-LIFT (in state)
Brain Injury Association of West Virginia
(304) 766-4892
(800) 356-6443 (in state)
Brain Injury Association of Wisconsin
(414) 271-7463
(800) 882-9282 (in state)
Brain Injury Association of Wyoming
(307) 473-1767
(800) 643-6457 (in state)

Affliliates

Alaska Head Injury Foundation
(907) 337-1441
Brain Association of Dallas
(214) 426-4444

Brain Injury Association of Washington, DC
(202) 877-1464
Long Island Head Injury Association
(516) 543-2245
Brain Injury Association of the Mid-South — Memphis, TN
(901) 452-3035
Northern Nevada Head Injury Association
(702) 828-7171
Brain Injury Association of Southern Nevada
(702) 454-7666
Newport Traumatic Brain Injury Association
(401) 847-2085
Pacific Head Injury Association Honolulu, HI
(808) 941-0372
South Dakota Brain Injury Association
(605) 229-2177
Brain Injury Association of Texas Gulf Coast Area
(713) 521-1880

On-Line Information

On-line information and support groups can be found at the following Web sites:

http://www.driveninc.com/
~jlyon/tbi.html
http://www.tbi.org
http://www.cai.net/naric
http://www.pacer.org
* http://unix.worldpath.net/
~rboyce/biahome.html

* This site is in the process of moving to the following address:
http://www.biausa.org/

Comments or questions for the authors may be sent via e-mail to the following internet address:

BrainInj@erols.com

ABOUT THE AUTHORS

Patt Abrahamson is a parent, guardian, and primary caretaker of her 46-year old son who has a brain injury. She has hosted a radio show and written a regular newspaper column dealing with social issues and topics of interest to older Americans. She has served as a Republican Party chairperson and has also co-chaired congressional campaigns. She is a trained social worker, received a bachelor of social work degree with honors from 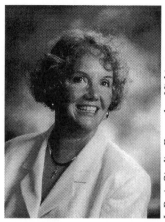 Northern Michigan University, and has been an advocate for the passage of the brain injury legislation in Congress. Winner of the Ms. Senior Michigan 1997 pageant, Patt lives in Escanaba, Michigan and North Fort Myers, Florida with her husband Gary Senior and their son Gary.

Patt wrote *Brain Injury: A Family Tragedy* in collaboration with her son, Jeffery Abrahamson. He is a legislative and regulatory specialist with Barnett & Sivon law firm in Washington, D.C. and has worked as a legislative aide on Capitol Hill as well as a lobbyist for Citicorp/Citibank. He received a B.A. in political science and economics from the University of Michigan and holds an M.B.A. in international business from George Washington University, where he also 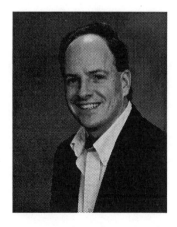 received a J.D. with honors. He has written articles for professional law journals and writes a monthly column for, and is an associate editor of, *Butterworths Journal of International Banking and Financial Law.* Jeffery lives in Burke, Virginia with his wife Peggy and daughter Mary Pat.